MIND YOUR BODY

MIND YOUR BODY

A SEXUAL HEALTH

AND WELLNESS

GUIDE FOR WOMEN

Beth Howard

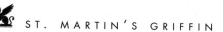 ST. MARTIN'S GRIFFIN ❧ NEW YORK

MIND YOUR BODY. Copyright © 1998 by Beth Howard. Printed in the United States of America. No part of this book may be used or reproduced in any manner whatsoever without written permission except in the case of brief quotations embodied in critical articles or reviews. For information, address St. Martin's Press, 175 Fifth Avenue, New York, N.Y. 10010.

DESIGN BY MAUREEN TROY

Library of Congress Cataloging-in-Publication Data

Howard, Beth.
    Mind your body : a sexual health and wellness guide for women / by Beth Howard.
        p.   cm.
    Includes bibliographical references.
    ISBN 0-312-18767-X
    1. Women—Health and hygiene.   2. Women—Sexual behavior.   3. Gynecology—Popular works.   I. Title.
RG121.H816   1998
613.9'54—dc21   98-13030
                                                                      CIP

First St. Martin's Griffin Edition: August 1998

10   9   8   7   6   5   4   3   2   1

To my grandfather,
Samuel L. Crow, M.D.,
whose dedication to healing was an inspiration
to everyone who knew him

Acknowledgments

I owe my warmest gratitude to the many researchers, physicians, nurse practitioners, and other health professionals who contributed their expertise and knowledge to this book. In particular I wish to thank Donna Shoupe, M.D., Felicia Stewart, M.D., Lauri J. Romanzi, M.D., Ellis Quinn Youngkin, Ph.D., R.N.C., Carol L. Otis, M.D., and Susan Tew.

This book was a true collaboration that began with an animated conversation between myself, my agent, Regula Noetzli, and my editor, Heather Jackson, in Grand Central Station, a place that for me has always symbolized new beginnings. Without their input, enthusiasm, and expert guidance, this book would never have been written.

I also wish to express my affection and gratitude to my friends and colleagues, particularly my good friend Kalia Doner, whose knowledge and encouragement were instrumental at every step of this adventure. Linda Marsa, Rebecca Norris, and Elizabeth M. Howard also shared their insights and support.

I am indebted to my editors at various magazines, particularly Elena Rover, Dana Points, and Paula Derrow, whose assignments helped shape the book. I also thank my pals at *Shape*—Peg Moline, Barbara Harris, Jenna McCarthy, Nancy Gottesman, and Carol Jacobs. For her support and encouragement in the end game, I offer my heartfelt appreciation to Clare McHugh, editor-in-chief of *New Woman* magazine. Special thanks also go to Marc Resnick at St. Martin's, who helped keep things on track, as well as to researchers Anne Gilbert, Lynda Liu, and Kelli Stauning.

I owe an enormous debt to Ken Goldstein, who gave me the tools and the courage to tackle science and health writing at the Columbia University Graduate School of Journalism.

Mark Zink read every page of this manuscript, offering uncommonly helpful suggestions, while maintaining his good humor—and also managed to keep me happy and well-fed. Barbara C. Rivers provided the love and support that only a mother can give—along with her extraordinary eye for detail. My sister, Judith H. Tompkins, generously compiled the bibliography.

Lastly, I thank my dear friend Jeanne Feeney—dancer, teacher, and healer—who first inspired me to think of my own body in a more positive and healthful way.

Contents

Contents

Preface

A small town in North Carolina is the last place you'd expect to find a gynecologist who specializes in straight talk about sex and sexual health. But this description fits Dr. Trent Busby, who retired in 1990 and died a few months later in Salisbury, North Carolina. Dr. Busby started practicing gynecology in 1953 and oversaw my mother's care when she moved to town as a young bride in the mid-1950s, delivering her first two children—my older sister and myself. Years later this quirky doctor was to become my first gynecologist.

Trent Busby was no Marcus Welby. Blustery in nature, with a complexion to match, he was wry, opinionated, and sometimes disconcertingly frank—traits often considered unbecoming to a physician. My mother disliked him at first. Her antipathy faded, however, when he remained at the hospital throughout the long hours of her troubled first labor and together (dads were not welcome in the labor room then) they delivered my sister. She remained his faithful patient for years, even traveling back to Salisbury for her annual exams after moving to a city an hour's drive away.

Studies show that doctors do not talk to their patients about sexually related matters because they fear offending them. In fact, there's evidence that physicians don't take vaginal health seriously, sometimes even ignoring the signs of common infections unless patients complain.

This was not true of Dr. Busby. Long before the breast cancer movement made the notion of becoming a partner in one's own health a popular idea, he came to the examining table with strong convictions about having informed patients. He took the risk of being rebuked by "holier-than-thou Victorian prudes," as he called them, asking the questions that needed to be asked in order to give women appropriate care. He railed against such practices as douching and using vaginal deodorants. In a small Southern town where manners and modesty prevailed, it was an uphill battle. Studies now confirm that douching leads to greater rates of pelvic inflammatory disease, which can impair a woman's fertility, and deodorant sprays increase the risk of developing ovarian cancer. Dr. Busby saw what feminine hygiene products did to healthy vaginas and appealed to women to "be good to their bodies," which later became the name of a book he wrote. Drawing waiting lists at the Rowan County Library for months, the book was an entertaining digest of Dr. Busby's opinions and pet peeves that, according to the *Salisbury Post,* "candidly addressed the delicate subjects that women were most curious about but dared not discuss."

Dr. Busby didn't judge his patients, and they didn't feel judged. And so he attracted plenty of women who, like me, discovered that his office was a safe place to ask awkward questions—and get straight answers and sound advice.

Unfortunately, few women have such an option when they seek gynecological care today. For one thing, there simply isn't time for the kind of thoroughness Dr. Busby provided. This is particularly true under HMOs and similar health plans, which allot a set amount of time to all patients, regardless of their individual needs. But more important, many physicians remain unwilling to drop the cloak of privacy and clue women in to the truths about their bodies and their health. Women pay the price for this lack of frank talk with contraceptive failures, health-threatening infections, and unfulfilling sex lives.

For these reasons, it is critical for women to take control of their sexual health. This book is intended to be a handbook for women who want to become knowledgeable about their bodies and stay healthy. It may also serve as a guide for a discussion with your gynecological or general health-care provider. The more you know before you go into the doctor's office, the better able you will be to ask for the care you need, forestall serious health problems, and, as Dr. Busby would say, "be good to your body."

Introduction

by Lauri J. Romanzi, M.D., FACOG

Mind Your Body is a thorough, thoughtful, educational, and entertaining book on issues of sexuality that affect the quality of life for women and men. In today's health-care environment, all of us are expected to be our own health advocates. This creates an exciting opportunity to educate ourselves and actively participate in our individual health-care issues, rather than relying solely on the "advice of experts." On the other hand, the stress of deciphering complex medical technology and the (now) competing interests of patients, doctors, hospitals, and insurers is often a less-than-positive experience. *Mind Your Body* is a reference guide that is both wide in scope and wise in content. From menarche to menopause, this guide to sexuality and sexual health answers health questions from a balanced perspective, allowing the reader to engage in information in a fashion which, as a physician, I believe will enhance the doctor-patient relationship.

Although geared to women (who are the traditional health-care brokers in their relationships with others), this is not a book "for girls only." Issues of contraception, sexually transmitted diseases, erotica, and sexual dysfunction are presented in a gender-balanced fashion. As a physician, I have found these topics to be tender interrelated areas, which patients share with me only after I have passed each woman's personal litmus test of compassion. This very appropriate screening tool is threatened in today's world of medicine, in which doctors are molded to think of patients not as individuals but as grouped "subscriber panels," with emphasis on "volume" and "efficiency," resulting in larger and larger numbers of patient visits per day than ever before. If medicine was a boutique business in the past, it is now rapidly transforming into a whole warehouse industry. This triage mentality may be cost effective (translate: profitable) in some regards, but it simply does not leave enough time for fine-tuning the intimacy of traditional doctor-patient relationships, which are operating in a large margin of deficit in this era of managed care. *Mind Your Body* reminds us all that quality-of-life issues and the interconnected facets of health, perception, and knowledge all impact on our well-being. These issues are as legitimate as chest pain and cancer and require as much priority, both in the health-care "market" and in the doctor's office. By providing concise, current reporting, *Mind Your Body* will encourage discourse in these neglected areas.

Even in the best of environments, sexual health–related issues remain difficult topics for many patients. While pertinent in the intimate moments of our lives, they can somehow seem less urgent, or simply too embarrassing, to dissect during an appointment with a doctor, nurse, or midwife in the middle of a busy week. *Mind Your Body* helps doctor and patient by allowing this intimate discussion to begin at a point of greater patient knowledge. Knowledge minimizes confusion and increases confidence. It also gives the patient a reference to review alone or with her family once our discussion takes place.

All aspects of health may ultimately impact on sexuality, for both women and men. *Mind Your Body* addresses this often neglected concept in a timely and balanced way.

Finally, lest a physician's recommendation bode poorly on anticipated reading pleasure, let me be the first to assure one and all that this book is as tasteful and humorous as it is instructive and factual.

MIND YOUR BODY

1 | Introduction: The Sexual Health Information Gap

"It's the last taboo we face in medicine."
"It's like the Arctic—we have no knowledge."
"It's a forgotten area."

These statements and many similar ones—pronounced by experts who were interviewed for this book—do not involve a rare disease, delivery of health to the poor, or the complexities of molecular biology. They actually concern different areas of women's sexual health. Even in the 90s, gynecological and sexual concerns are a frontier of medical research, victims of the same attitudes and taboos that keep them mysteries in the minds of women themselves.

Sexual health concerns still meet with embarrassment in labs, hospitals, and medical schools, so it is little wonder that there is a sizable sexual health information gap between doctor and patient. This gap is not good for women or society. Consider these facts:

- In a recent Gallup survey, nearly 50 percent of physicians reported that they did not treat the most common vaginal infection, bacterial vaginosis (BV), if patients didn't complain of symptoms—even when the doctors found evidence of it. Now it turns out that BV may not be so benign: Researchers have linked it to greater rates of preterm birth, among other problems.
- Nearly half of women patients mistakenly believe that they are being screened for all manner of infections when they undergo their annual gynecological exam, according to a recent Kaiser Family Foundation survey. Many women also err in thinking that the Pap smear picks up diseases other than cervical cancer.
- When asked to name STDs, only 25 percent of women mentioned chlamydia, by far the most prevalent STD, which can lead to pelvic inflammatory disease (PID) and impair fertility. Making matters worse, doctors do not routinely screen for chlamydia despite the 4 million annual cases that push chlamydia into the epidemic category—and up to 80 percent of women with the STD have no symptoms.

The sexual health information gap also shows up in more routine areas, such as contraceptive concerns. Almost half of unintended pregnancies each year occur with women who are *using* birth control. Yet contraceptive experts agree that most available methods of birth control are extremely effective at preventing pregnancy if used correctly and consistently.

Clearly something important is being lost in the communication between doctor and patient. For example, most gynecologists know about "after-the-fact" means of avoiding pregnancy when accidents occur, but the majority mention it to patients only if women bring it up. Knowledge of safe and effective emergency contraception could reduce the number of unplanned pregnancies each year by 1.7 million and the number of abortions by 800,000, according to the authors of *Contraceptive Technology*, the sexual health authority for health-care practitioners.

Few doctors teach women basic facts about female physiology, including information that could help them more easily avoid pregnancy. (Often this information is lacking from physicians' own medical educations.) For example, the cervix changes shape at the time of ovulation, becoming elongated and more open. It makes sense to have a diaphragm or cervical cap fitted at this time in the cycle to optimize the device's effectiveness, but providers rarely emphasize this important point.

This book is intended to help fill the sexual health information gap by providing up-to-date information about sexual anatomy, function, and expression. The goal is to keep you healthy and to help you make sex more gratifying and meaningful. Think of it as foreplay in the broadest sense.

Chapter 2 lays the groundwork for general sexual wellness. It invites you to get to know your unique sexual landscape and become a partner in your own health. Do you exercise and eat vegetables? Your sexual health deserves the same commitment as your physical well-being. Adopting an assertive posture toward your sexual health empowers you to prevent many physical problems that can mar your life and your intimate experiences. (This section also includes basic breast-care information.)

Chapter 3 gives you additional tools for troubleshooting by describing the cyclical nature of feminine physiology, the basics of ovulation and menstruation, and the causes and cures of common problems that frequently crop up as part of these processes. This section explores menstruation myths as a means of challenging women to rethink their attitudes about such female phenomena. The idea is to begin to see your body as an ally, not an enemy, in the striving to live well and succeed. An attitude adjustment should pay off nicely in both the bedroom and the doctor's office.

Chapter 4 prepares women for choosing a method of contraception that suits their needs by outlining each method's advantages and disadvantages. It also includes critical information to help you improve the efficacy of your birth control. The more you know about your contraception, the more confident you will be of its ability to protect you against pregnancy and/or disease—and the better your time spent between the sheets. Additionally, this chapter includes information on emergency birth control and contraceptive advances to look for in the coming years.

Sexuality itself is the subject of Chapter 5, which allows that seeking sexual fulfillment is far from a frivolous pursuit. It is a basic human need. Culled from the scientific literature, this chapter summarizes the research on sexual response and behavior and explores trends in sexual expression. The ideas presented may help give your sex life new dimensions.

Chapter 6 examines the ailments, attitudes, and emotions that can spoil sex. Beginning with a discussion of our remarkable vaginal ecology (and prescriptions for maintaining vaginal health), this section details the sources, symptoms, and remedies of common infections and sex-stopping conditions; prescription and nonprescription medications that can interfere with intimacy; and the causes and cures of sexual dysfunction. The chapter features the sex therapist's "tool box"—some proven therapeutic methods that can be used to tackle sex-related woes. This section ends with some insights about sexual coercion and ideas about avoiding confusing sexual situations.

A discussion of sexually transmitted diseases (STDs) makes up Chapter 7. This chapter describes these sexual scourges and emphasizes why women in particular should educate themselves about these diseases, as women are more vulnerable than men to infection and the long-term consequences of STDs. The chapter concludes with detailed guidelines for safe sex and new advances in HIV testing that should help women to stay healthy—and happy—in bed.

Chapter 8 explores sexual health and aging, and includes an update on research related to hormone replacement therapy. Lastly, the book answers frequently *unasked* questions about sexual health and provides a resource section for further exploration.

Mind Your Body should help women:

- develop greater body awareness
- understand the limitations of their birth control method and how to maximize its effectiveness

- understand the risks of sexual activity and how to minimize exposure to infectious diseases
- ask for tests they need and question treatments that may be unnecessary
- overcome shame and embarrassment about their bodies
- achieve greater health and sexual well-being.

2 | Sexual Geography

The Feminine Landscape

Vagina. This simple three-syllable word is no tongue twister—but it often leaves even the bold among us sputtering.

And it's not just talking about vaginas that makes people nervous. A surprising number of women can't bring themselves to look at their own sexual anatomy. The vagina is the locus of our most profound feelings and attitudes about intimacy. No wonder it is shrouded in mystery and shame—or that the men in our lives often know their way around our bodies better than we do. (Of course, there is the practical issue of access: While women have to make an effort to get a look at their sexual equipment, men can survey their own by simply glancing in a mirror.) Not surprisingly, many women ignore matters related to their sexual anatomy and function.

But medicine is also guilty of keeping women's sexual anatomy under wraps. Research on the vagina and the vulva—the external genitalia—is nearly nonexistent. And medical training is notoriously scanty. "Some physicians learn how to do a pelvic exam from a video," says R. Allen Lawhead, M.D., chairman of the Department of Obstetrics and Gynecology at Georgia Baptist Medical Center in Atlanta.

Even the medical specialists have a history of limiting their scope. Gynecologists tend to focus on the cervix and internal reproductive organs; urologists, on urinary tract problems. Most dermatologists stop short of the pubic area. That leaves a sizable area of neglect. "The vagina is a forgotten area for all medical specialists," says Peter Lynch, M.D., chairman of the Department of Dermatology at the University of California at Davis. "When you add the sexual taboos, it has been virtually ignored."

Add to this women's historic neglect of their bodies and you've got the setup for a stalemate: Doctors don't ask about sexually related matters, and women don't tell.

Women pay a high price for this privacy. At its worst, physician and patient

Your vaginal "barrel"—as it is sometimes inelegantly called by scientists—has remarkable flexibility. It measures approximately 2½ to 3 inches wide by 3½ to 4 inches long. The surface has ridges, called rugae, which make it appear and feel corrugated, like an accordion. The rugae grip the penis during sex. They also help the vagina balloon and lengthen to accommodate an erect penis or a fetus during childbirth. After repeated births or menopause, the rugae gradually disappear.

In the 1960s, William Masters, M.D., and Virginia Johnson, the famed sex research team, discovered that the vaginal walls are ingeniously engineered for sex. The lining, or epithelium, appears to perspire during sexual arousal, producing the lubrication handy for intercourse. Previously researchers believed that special glands performed this function. This sexual "sweat" is not to be confused with cervical mucus, which can be felt at the

miss early signs of disease. Even at best, many women suffer in silence, too embarrassed to complain about bodily woes that are diminishing their health and their happiness in bed.

When it comes to your sexual health, what you don't know *can* hurt you. That's why you owe it to yourself to end the stalemate.

The first step is to get acquainted with your body. "If you don't know what you look like, then how are you going to know everything is okay?" asks Debra Gussman, M.D., a Denver gynecologist. The more you know about yourself, the better able you will be to notice signs of disease before they develop into serious problems and the more empowered you will feel to ask for care when you need it. By learning about your sexual anatomy, you may also help your doctor understand the benefits of having an educated patient.

Sexual Anatomy 101

External Organs

(The external genitalia are collectively called the *vulva*.)

- The *mons veneris* is the soft, fleshy mound, covered by pubic hair, that protects the internal organs.
- The *labia majora* are the protruding outer lips that provide padding and protection to the vaginal and urinary openings.
- The *labia minora* are the inner lips of soft skin that covers the vagina. During sexual arousal they become engorged with blood and fill out to accommodate the penis. Both inner and outer lips have abundant nerve endings and are responsive to pleasurable sensations as well as pain.
- The two inner lips join to form the *clitoral hood*, which protects the clitoris.
- The *clitoris* is the organ responsible for a woman's orgasm. It fills with blood during sexual arousal and becomes firm and erect, like a penis. It lies beneath the clitoral hood above the urinary opening. (*See Chapter 5 for more on the clitoris.*)
- The *vestibule* is the area that lies inside and between the labia minora. The urethral opening is situated toward the front of the vestibule, and behind the urethral opening is the hymen, which partially covers the vagina. Opening into the vestibule are glands called Bartholin's glands, which secrete fluid during sexual arousal.

The Vulva

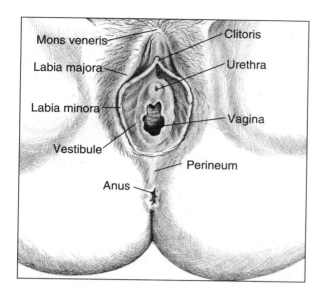

Mons veneris

Labia majora

Labia minora

Vestibule

Anus

Clitoris

Urethra

Vagina

Perineum

American College of Obstetricians and Gynecologists. *Diseases of the Vulva*. (Patient Education Pamphlet No. AP088.) Washington, D.C. © ACOG.

opening of the vagina, says Toni Weschler, M.P.H., author of *Taking Charge of Your Fertility*.

At menopause, the vagina changes due to declining estrogen levels. Both the vulva (the external genitalia) and the vagina become drier and less elastic, and the vagina begins to narrow and shorten in a process called *vaginal atrophy*. The vaginal walls also become thinner, retain less moisture, and are slower to lubricate. Estrogen replacement can reduce the severity of these changes. *(For more information, see "Hormone Therapy," page 189.)*

Internal Organs

- The *uterus* is a pear-shaped mass of muscle in the lower abdomen. Its main role is to shelter a growing fetus. It's connected to the fallopian tubes at the top, and narrows down into the cervix and vagina at the bottom.
- The *fallopian tubes* are about four to five inches long and transport eggs from the ovary to the uterus. When fertilization occurs, it happens about a third of the way into this journey.
- The *ovaries* are the two almond-shaped glands connected to the fallopian tubes. They contain up to a million eggs when we are born, and they produce estrogen and progesterone throughout our reproductive lives.
- The *endometrium* is the blood-rich lining of the uterus that builds up during ovulation in preparation for pregnancy. When conception doesn't occur, it is shed each month as menstrual blood.

Female Sexual Anatomy

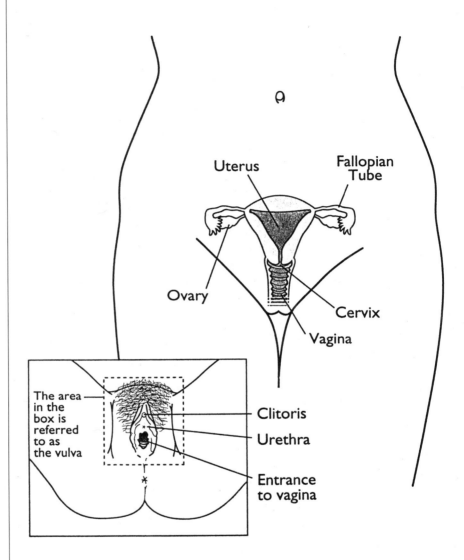

AVCS International © 1992 by David Rosenzweig

- The *cervix* is the lower opening of the uterus. It is visible during a gynecological exam, and it can be felt with your fingertips at the end of the vagina. The tiny opening in the center is called the *cervical os*.
- The *vagina* is the muscular tube that connects the uterus to the outside of the body. Menstrual blood leaves the body via the vagina.

A Vagina by Any Other Name . . .

In the fall of 1996 the New York theater scene witnessed a provocative new play called *The Vagina Monologues*. But notice of this funny and unflinching exploration of women's attitudes toward their bodies barely made it into the venerable *New York Times*. The word *vagina*, the newspaper deemed, was not fit to print.

Vagina may not be a four-letter word, but using it is a good way to make people squirm—which is one reason they've come up with so many creative substitutions, according to Eve Ensler, author of *The Vagina Monologues*:

"In Great Neck they call it Pussycat—a woman's mother used to tell her, 'Don't wear panties underneath your pajamas; you need to air out your pussycat.' In Westchester they call it a pooki; in New Jersey, a twat. There's Powderbox, Derriere, a Poochi, a Peepe, a Poopelu, a Pal and a Piche, Tuckas, Toadie, Dee Dee, Nishi, Dignity, Coochi Snatcher, Cooter, Labbe, Gladys Seagleman, VA, Wee Wee, Horsespot, Nappy Dugout, Mongo, a Pajama, Fannyboo, Mushmellow, a Ghoulie, Possible, Tamale, Tottita, Connie, a Mimi in Miami, Split Knish in Philadelphia, and Schmende in the Bronx.

"I am worried about vaginas."

—from *The Vagina Monologues*, by Eve Ensler

The Vulvar Self-Exam

A Guided Tour of the Feminine Landscape

The vulvar self-exam, or VSE, is a monthly check of the vulva—the external genitalia. It's simple to perform and can be coupled with your monthly breast self-exam.

"The vulvar self-exam does not cost the health-care system or women anything, and its benefits are priceless," says R. Allen Lawhead, M.D.

Vulvar vigilance pays off in several ways: Women who perform the

PRIVATE VIEWING

You'd expect a book with thirty-two close-up color shots of women's genitals to be a big hit with men. But *Femalia*, published in 1994 by Down There Press, is really intended for women—especially those women who mistakenly believe that their own sex organs are somehow not quite up to snuff.

The reason for the book is simple: Unlike men, most women don't have opportunities to compare themselves to other women. This simple, textless book addresses women's insecurities by celebrating the different sizes and wide variety of labia, introitus (vaginal entrance), and clitorises. To order a copy of *Femalia*, contact Good Vibrations/Down There Press, 938 Howard Street, Suite 101, San Francisco, CA 94103; 415-974-8990.

VSE regularly can detect common skin disorders and viral infections such as genital warts and herpes and get treated earlier. The self-exam can also detect vulvar cancer, a rare but deadly cancer that in later phases may require disfiguring surgery. "Thousands of women would benefit from this," Lawhead says. "Over 95 percent of women with vulvar cancer have had symptoms months to years before they were diagnosed." The good news: You can almost always see cancerous lesions in the early stages, and they can almost always be cured without extreme measures.

Here's how to do it:

1. Sit down on a soft surface, such as a bed, upholstered chair, or carpet. (If you are pregnant or obese, or if you have a debilitating condition like arthritis, you can lie with your head propped up by a pillow or stand with one leg on a stool.)
2. Hold a mirror in one hand and use the other to expose the tissue of the vulva.
3. Make sure you have a good source of light. Then examine—by looking *and* touching—the following areas:

- The mons veneris (the area around the pubic bone, which is covered with pubic hair)
- The clitoris and the area that surrounds it (gently retract the hood to get a good view)
- The labia majora (the fleshy, hair-covered outer lips of the vagina)
- The labia minora (the inner folds of skin on either side of the vaginal opening)
- The vestibule (or vaginal opening), where the labia minora meet at the bottom
- The perineum, the space between the vagina and the anus (women who have given birth sometimes have an episiotomy scar).

Basically, you're looking for any change or new growth, including new moles, warts, or other growths; changes in skin color, especially white, red, or darkened areas; sores and ulcers; and areas that are inflamed, irritated, or itching. Unless they were caused by a simple injury, any changes should be reported to your health-care provider. Taking responsibility for your health in this way will enhance the quality of care you get from your health-care provider and help keep you in charge of your sexual health.

Back in the Stirrups Again: The Basic Gynecological Exam

Power to the Patient

You're flat on your back in a flimsy paper gown, flesh against a cold examining table, your legs propped up in stirrups. There are few times when a woman feels quite as vulnerable as when she is waiting for a pelvic examination. If you're tense and flustered, you're likely to feel greater discomfort when the doctor begins the exam or forget important things you wanted to ask about.

There are many things you can do to make yourself more comfortable, however, to overcome your sense of vulnerability as well as optimize your time with your health-care provider. If you want to be a partner with your provider, you will have to take some control. You can do this starting with your next physical. Here's how:

- Ask to start the exam in your provider's office while you are still dressed. This is your opportunity to let your provider know any concerns you have about your health or to ask any questions. It is easier to bring up awkward and embarrassing issues when you are fully clothed. Many providers automatically start appointments in the office. "I never examine anybody until I can talk to them first," says Ellis Quinn Youngkin, Ph.D., R.N.C., a women's health nurse-practitioner and coordinator of the Graduate Program at the College of Nursing, Florida Atlantic University, in Boca Raton.

- If you are particularly nervous, consider bringing a friend to your exam. Many providers will allow you to have someone in the room with you, but you should ask first.

- Come prepared with a list of your concerns. Studies have shown that people who make lists before visits are less anxious when they leave the doctor's office. Be prepared to write down the answers to your questions, so you can refer to them later.

- Bring along a pair of warm socks to wear during the exam.

- If you are sexually active, you may need to be tested for chlamydia and gonorrhea—and you may have to ask for these tests. Although the Centers for Disease Control (CDC) recommends routine screenings for these STDs, little more than half of women are offered these tests as a matter of course. If your doctor doesn't perform these tests as part of routine screenings, ask for them. Chlamydia and gonorrhea, which are often symptomless, can lead to pelvic inflammatory disease (PID) and if left unchecked can impair your ability to have children. *(For more on chlamydia, see page 162.)*

- Make sure your provider performs a breast exam. A smart way to bring it up: Ask for a review of your own technique. The American College of Obstetricians and Gynecologists recommends a breast exam by a doctor once a year. Until recently, breast exams weren't a mandatory part of gynecological training, however, so some doctors are not skilled in the technique.
- Urinate before and after your pelvic exam. Research from the University of Illinois College of Medicine has shown that some women get a urinary tract infection after their checkup, probably because bacteria are inadvertently pushed into the urethra, according to Jeffrey D. Tiemstra, M.D., director of family medicine for the University of Illinois in Urbana.

Note: If your doctor resists your attempts to be involved in your own health care, it may be time to switch to a provider who is more open to your participation. Many doctors and other health-care providers welcome it. Nurse-practitioners with special training in women's health and midwives are often particularly receptive to your input.

Taking the Pain Out of Pelvic Exams

After your provider examines your vulva—your external genitalia—for discharge or signs of sexually transmitted diseases (STDs) and other problems, the next steps are the insertion of the speculum and preparation of the Pap smear, when your provider takes samples of cells from your cervix to test for signs of disease. The speculum is an instrument that opens the vagina so that the practitioner can get a good look. (You'll feel some pressure as it is put into place.) During the pelvic and rectal exams, your provider inspects your internal organs visually and manually. Marcia Szmania Davis, M.S., a women's health-care nurse-practitioner at Virginia Commonwealth University in Richmond, offers these tips for staying relaxed and comfortable.

What to Do
- Imagine that you have five-pound weights resting on your knees. "A lot of the discomfort comes from the fact that women are pressing so hard on the speculum," Davis says. "If you let your legs go loose, it helps."

- Practice abdominal breathing. Rest both hands across your mid-abdomen. Take a deep breath. As you inhale, watch your hands separate slightly then come together again on the exhale. Focusing on your breathing will keep you distracted and make you less likely to tense up.
- Think about what your body feels like the first thing in the morning—before you get out of bed. Try to shift into this super-relaxed mode on the exam table.

What Not to Do

- Don't raise your head or put your hands behind your head. Lifting your head has the same effect as a crunch: It tenses your abdominal muscles—just when you need to relax them.
- Don't endure pain. If you feel extreme discomfort, tell your practitioner. She should be able to alleviate your pain by adjusting her position. And telling her about any pain you have can alert her to hidden health problems.
- Don't be alarmed if you bleed a little after your examination. That's normal.

The Pap Smear

Fifty years ago, cervical cancer was the leading cause of cancer death in women. No more, thanks to a simple test called the Pap smear. Developed by George Papanicolaou, M.D., it is responsible for reducing deaths from cervical cancer by 70 percent since it was introduced in the early 1940s.

In spite of the Pap smear's excellent track record, many women have lost faith in the test in recent years due to tragic cases in which smears were misread. In 1995, Karin Smith, a Milwaukee accountant, died from cervical cancer despite having had three Pap smears, each of which was interpreted as normal. Smith's lawyers argued that the lab her HMO used for Pap smear testing processed more slide samples than could be reasonably read by lab technicians. The HMO was found guilty of reckless homicide.

It's good to know that federal law now limits cytologists—the technicians who read the slides—to a hundred slides per day. After a flurry of media reports exposing inferior lab practices in the late 1980s, Congress passed the Clinical Laboratory Improvement Amendments (CLIA) with regulations concerning training of technicians who process the slides, their workloads, and their accuracy levels.

PROFILE OF A PAP
SMEAR

Main Claim to Fame: Single-handedly responsible for reducing cervical cancer death rate by 70 percent since the early 1940s.

The Basics: With the speculum in place, cells are gently scraped from both the outer part of the cervix and the cervical canal. (Don't worry. You'll only feel a pinch.) The cells are smeared onto a slide and fixed with a substance that preserves the sample until it is sent to the lab. There, the slides are examined under a microscope to identify abnormal cells.

Tools of the Trade: Practitioners use different implements for obtaining cell samples—wooden or plastic "spatulas," small wandlike brushes, and cotton swabs. Studies have shown that a cytobrush, which looks like a mascara wand, is more effective than cotton swabs at obtaining a good smear.

When You Should Get It: If you are sexually active or have reached the age of

The bad news about the Pap smear is that up to 20 percent of those taken from women with cancerous or precancerous cells are wrongly reported as normal. These so-called false negatives can hinder prompt diagnosis and proper treatment. The good news: If you get a Pap smear regularly, your chances of getting false negatives drop significantly.

Getting a Pap smear is more important than ever. Knowing the facts about it—and the ways we ourselves can improve it—should help reduce fears.

The Curable Cancer?

Luckily, cases of extreme negligence like Karin Smith's are rare, and they don't negate the value of the Pap smear. In fact, many experts believe cervical cancer could be virtually eliminated as a cause of death if all women got screened regularly.

Cervical cancer develops slowly—though often without symptoms until it is advanced. Currently about five thousand women die from it each year. Experts have linked the disease to a common sexually transmitted virus called human papilloma virus (HPV), which causes genital warts. Researchers don't know exactly how HPV leads to cancer, but they believe it is related to the type of HPV a woman has. (More than eighty different types have been identified, so far.) It's important to remember, however, that most women with HPV will not get cervical cancer.

According to Ralph M. Richart, M.D., professor of pathology, obstetrics and gynecology at Columbia Presbyterian Medical Center in New York City, certain types of HPV are associated with cervical cancer. These include types 16, 18, 31, 33, 35, 51, 52, and 56. Because some types are more dangerous than others, some doctors have begun typing women with HPV to determine whether they have one of the HPV viruses associated with cervical cancer. In the future, women with these types may be watched more carefully than those with less suspicious types of HPV.

To that end, medical supply companies are now marketing HPV typing test kits, which identify the DNA structure of the virus, thus telling practitioners whether the virus a woman carries is likely to develop into cancer. Some medical researchers have proposed a new screening regimen that would use both Pap smears and HPV typing, making treatment decisions more appropriate. Those women who are found to have HPV types associated with cervical cancer would be monitored more closely. Doctors would test them more frequently for precancerous changes and thus be able to treat them aggressively when changes are detected.

Interpreting the Pap Smear

The Pap smear is not a pass-fail test, which can be frustrating for both providers and patients. In some cases the sample was inadequate: It had too few cervical cells for the lab technician to make a judgment, or the cervical cells were obscured by other cells, say from blood or infection. Then the test has to be repeated.

The problem arises when the cells on your Pap smear don't look normal, though they aren't clearly cancerous, either. Often doctors take a wait-and-see approach with such results, having you return for a follow-up smear in a few months' time. Much of the time these ambiguous results will return to normal on the follow-up test, though a small number of these will turn out to be cancerous. Don't panic if you get an abnormal result—chances are good you do not have cancer.

Although the number of abnormal Pap smears is increasing, it does not mean that cancer rates are rising. It may be a consequence of a new Pap smear classification reporting system, called the Bethesda System, which was instituted to make Pap smear readings more meaningful. It characterizes cell changes and offers guidelines for treatment of abnormal conditions.

"Because of the change in reporting, women are more likely to be told they have a borderline smear," says Dr. Richart. "They need not panic because most aren't anything to worry about. But women do need to pay attention to the results and be evaluated appropriately."

The Bethesda System classifies Pap smears in seven broad categories. Here's what you should know about them:

Unsatisfactory

What it means: Not enough cells were sampled or the cells were taken from the wrong part of the cervix.

Follow-up: You must have another Pap smear within three to six months.

Normal

What it means: All the cells in an adequate sample appeared normal.

Follow-up: None. Mark your calendar to have another exam in one year.

eighteen, the American College of Obstetricians and Gynecologists and the American Cancer Institute recommend getting a Pap test and pelvic examination annually. If you have three consecutive years of satisfactory, normal readings, your doctor may suggest you have the screening less frequently. However, you should definitely get a yearly test if you smoke, if you have more than one sex partner, if you have HPV, if you have any sexually transmitted diseases (STDs), or if you are infected with HIV, the virus that causes AIDS.

Reassuring Fact #1: Only about 20 percent of cases in which smears indicated the presence of precancerous cells develop into cancer.

Reassuring Fact #2: You are more than likely to get accurately diagnosed, if you get regular tests. On average 20 percent of Pap smears are false negatives, but if two Pap smears are performed within a few months, the rate drops to 4 percent. If there are three Pap smears, the rate drops to a nearly negligible .8 percent.

Several recent technological
advances are expected to
maximize your chances of
getting an accurate Pap
smear:

After viewing the Pap
smear slides once, cytologists—who are specially
trained to identify defective
cells in slides—typically rescreen about 10 percent of
the samples. The *Autopap
300 System* makes it possible to rescreen all the samples. Using sophisticated
imaging technologies developed by the Department of
Defense, it picks out 10 to
20 percent of the most
suspicious-looking smears for
a second look by a cytologist. The manufacturers of
Autopap claim it will find
five times the number of abnormal samples as a manual
screen.

The *Papnet System* also
rescreens Pap smears that a
cytologist has found to be
normal. It selects the 128
most suspicious cells or cell
clusters from each Pap
smear. They are recorded on
a large color video monitor

Benign Reactive

What it means: May indicate the presence of an infection, such as a yeast infection, or a bacterial disease such as chlamydia.

Follow-up: Treat the problem and repeat the test in three to six months.

Atypical Squamous Cells of Undetermined Significance (ASCUS)

What it means: This is the gray area of Pap smear readings. Cells show some evidence of change but are not clearly cancerous. "We're not sure if they're abnormal or not, but they don't look quite right," says Dr. Youngkin.

Follow-up: You may wait for three or six months and have the Pap test repeated. Sometimes the changes go away. Sometimes, however, your practitioner may perform a procedure that magnifies the view of the cervix (using a technique called colposcopy) and takes a small sample (a biopsy) from any areas that look suspicious. If the biopsy is normal, your doctor will probably repeat the test in six months. If the sample shows a precancer or a cancer, you will have more tissue removed. You may have some pain or discharge for a few days after the procedure. You will have more frequent follow-up Pap smears for a while until you have three consecutive normal smears, then you can return to your yearly routine.

Low-Grade Squamous Intraepithelial Lesions (LGSIL)

What it means: Also called dysplasia, these are cells that are slightly pre-cancerous or show signs of infection with HPV, the precursor to cervical cancer.

Follow-up: Same as ASCUS.

High-grade SIL (HGSIL)

What it means: Sample shows moderate to severe precancerous cells.

Follow-up: Same as ASCUS, though more aggressively treated and watched.

Squamous Cancer

What it means: Cells appear to be cancerous.

Follow-up: Same as above. This is a serious diagnosis. If the lesion is severe or persistent, the uterus may eventually be removed.

Seven Steps to a Better Pap Test

1. Schedule your Pap smear at midcycle—about twelve to fourteen days before or after your period is a good rule of thumb. The presence of menstrual blood can obscure abnormal cells.
2. Don't put anything in the vagina for seventy-two hours before the exam. That means no vaginal medications, lubricants, douches, or contraceptive products—and no sexual intercourse.
3. Alert your physician to any abnormal vaginal discharge, which can compromise the test's accuracy. If necessary, reschedule the Pap portion of your exam when you are free from infection.
4. Ask your provider to use a cytobrush to obtain cell samples. Studies have shown it to be more effective in getting an adequate specimen.
5. Call the lab associated with your clinic or gynecologist and ask if it is certified by the American Society of Cytology or College of American Pathologists. Strongly consider finding a practitioner who works with a certified lab.
6. Don't assume that if you don't hear from your physician it means everything is fine. Always call to verify your results.
7. Ask that a copy of the lab's report be sent to you. This is your opportunity to verify the social security number and name to rule out the possibility of a mix-up with another patient. Also verify that the Pap test had an adequate specimen of cervical cells. Look for the words "optimal" or "adequate sample." If they do not appear on the report, the physician didn't get enough cells, and the test should be repeated.

for a second evaluation by the cytologist. Studies show that it picks up about one-third more abnormal cells initially missed by the first screening.

The *Thin Prep 2000 System* was designed to reduce the number of samples judged to be unreadable because of the presence of blood or mucus. The brush used to obtain the cell sample is rinsed in a vial with a preservative. Then the solution is sent to a lab where an instrument filters out contaminants. A thin layer of cells is applied to a slide for inspection.

Ask your health-care provider or the lab if it uses any of these technologies and request one of them if you are at increased risk for cervical cancer—or just want extra reassurance. Keep in mind that you will probably pay more for the added peace of mind, about forty dollars for the Autopap and Papnet technologies and another twenty dollars for Thin Prep.

Breast Health

As is true with other areas of women's sexual anatomy such as the vulva and the vagina, issues related to the breast are often sources of embarrassment and, consequently, neglect for many women. The fear of breast cancer is itself often an obstacle to good breast health. The consequences of failing to care for your breasts are potentially deadly.

Taking charge of your breasts is a critical component of sexual wellness with significant physical and emotional benefits. The first step is knowledge. Here are some common areas of concern:

Breast Pain

Sixty percent of women suffer from breast pain, or mastalgia, but a great many of them put up with it because they're too embarrassed to tell their doctors. Or they may ignore the pain, fearing that it is linked to cancer. If you suffer from breast pain, you should know that it is rarely associated with cancer, and there is much that can be done to ease your discomfort.

Breast pain has many causes, including normal life stages—such as the onset of puberty or menopause—PMS, pregnancy, engorgement of the breast following childbirth, and normal hormonal fluctuations. Breast pain is also a side effect of certain drugs such as digitalis preparations, aldomet, aldactone, certain diuretics, anadrol, and chlorpromazine.

Cyclical breast pain is tenderness or discomfort that is related to the menstrual cycle. Most women who suffer from this type of mastalgia have greater pain in one breast. Timing can vary: Some experience pain midcycle with ovulation, others are more sensitive just prior to their menstrual period.

Many women find relief from their symptoms through simple good-health measures, such as cutting back on caffeine, taking vitamin E supplements, and eating a low-fat diet. Some health practitioners advise their patients to take evening primrose oil daily in a dose of three grams. (This substance can cause miscarriage, however, so it should not be used by women who are pregnant or trying to conceive.) Your doctor may also prescribe drugs, including Danazol and bromocriptane.

Noncyclical breast pain occurs irregularly. Often women can pinpoint a specific site of pain. Burning pains around the nipple may result from dilation of the ducts. Other sources are more mysterious. Pain in the chest wall or spine can be caused by a certain type of arthritis, called costochondritis. Analgesic or nonsteriodal anti-inflammatory drugs can help ease the pain. Similarly, a pinched nerve in the neck can cause pain to radiate to the breast, in which case your doctor may prescribe analgesics and physiotherapy.

Breast Cancer

Nothing strikes fear in women like breast cancer, the most common cancer in women and the second deadliest one after lung cancer. Breast cancer strikes about 185,000 women each year, killing some 43,000.

The outlook for women with breast cancer has significantly brightened in recent years with improved and refined treatments. With early detection, most women who have breast cancer will not die from it, and in many cases, a woman's breast can be spared. The following facts underscore the importance of being alert to changes in your breasts and taking care of them:

- More than 80 percent of breast lumps are found to be benign, or noncancerous.
- More than 90 percent of women who find and treat breast cancer early are cancer free at five years.
- There are more than 1.6 million breast cancer survivors in the United States.

The information provided below is intended to help put breast cancer risk in perspective and provide information for preventing the occurrence of the disease as a part of general sexual health. There are several good resources that describe what a diagnosis of breast cancer means and that outline the treatment options if you have been diagnosed with this disease. (See Breast Cancer Resources, page 25.)

Breast Cancer Risk Factors

The following conditions and factors are associated with increased breast cancer incidence. Having one or more of these factors does not mean you will develop breast cancer, just that you have a somewhat greater risk for it.

Some factors you can control, others you cannot. Even if you have genetic risk factors, you may be able to influence your risk by compensating in those areas within your control.

- *Family history.* A mother, sister, or daughter has had the disease. Family risk is linked to two genes, BRCA1 and BRCA2, scientists say. Having the BRCA1 gene presents an 85 percent lifetime chance of developing breast cancer.
- *Atypical hyperplasia.* Premenopausal women diagnosed with this benign breast condition have an increased lifetime risk for developing breast cancer.
- *Late or no pregnancy/no breastfeeding.* A woman who has her first child after age thirty or who remains childless has a slightly increased risk over her lifetime. The protection kicks in with the first pregnancy carried to term. Breastfeeding appears to protect further against breast cancer.
- *Early menstruation/late menopause.* Both confer a slightly greater breast cancer risk. (Women who have a hysterectomy before age thirty-five have a decreased risk.)
- *Hormone replacement therapy/birth control pills.* Controversy continues about the role of estrogen in amplifying cancer risk; a recent meta-analysis of studies showed that birth control pills do not con-

19

fer a long-term breast cancer risk, according to researchers at Oxford University. *(See "Reconsidering the Pill," page 56.)* The jury is still out on whether taking HRT increases a woman's risk, but many researchers believe the risk is small.

- *Alcohol use.* A number of studies have linked alcohol intake (one or two drinks daily) with an increased risk.
- *Radiation therapy for Hodgkin's disease.* The cancer risk persists for ten years following the last treatment.
- *Age.* The older you are, the greater the chance for mutations that can trigger uncontrolled cell growth, the hallmark of cancer. Half of all breast cancers occur in women ages fifty to sixty-four, and 30 percent in women over seventy.
- *Obesity.* Carrying around as little as ten extra pounds increases your risk for developing breast cancer by almost 25 percent in your thirties, even more as you age.

RISK OF DEVELOPING BREAST CANCER IN THE NEXT YEAR

You've probably heard that one in eight women will develop cancer over her lifetime. But your cancer risk varies considerably depending on your age.

AGE	RISK
20 to 24	1 in 110,000
25 to 29	1 in 12,850
30 to 34	1 in 3,700
35 to 39	1 in 1,555
40 to 44	1 in 790
45 to 49	1 in 531
50 to 54	1 in 450
55 to 59	1 in 386
60 to 64	1 in 292
65 to 69	1 in 244
70 to 74	1 in 215
75 to 79	1 in 215

Source: National Cancer Institute

Breast Cancer Prevention

There's not much you can do about starting menstruation early or a family history of breast cancer. If you have any risk factors for breast cancer, it is particularly important to be vigilant about prevention and early detection. For instance, you can stay within a normal weight for your age by exercising and eating a low-fat diet, and you can limit your consumption of alcohol. Here are the current guidelines for prevention and early detection.

Regular Mammograms After Forty

Beginning at age forty, have a regular mammogram, or X ray of the breast, every year or two until the age of fifty, then have one annually. Researchers have been bickering about these points for a number of years. The debate has centered around whether women between the ages of forty and fifty should get mammograms regularly. In January 1997, an advisory panel of the National Institutes of Health (NIH) concluded that there was no data to support regular screenings for women in their forties. The American Cancer Society vehemently disagreed with the findings, strongly recommending that routine screening begin at age forty.

Proponents of the more vigilant approach cite this evidence: Of the new cases of breast cancer that will be diagnosed this year, 20 to 25 percent will be in women under fifty. Studies have shown a reduced mortality rate, perhaps as high as 30 percent, in women in this age group whose cancer was discovered through mammography. The value in the test increases as a woman nears fifty. Those who argue against regular screenings for women between forty and fifty cite the larger number of unnecessary biopsies, anxiety due to false alarms, and radiation risk from the test.

Controversies about how often and when to get a mammogram do not negate the value of the test and the importance of regular screening, especially if you have a family history of the disease. If you are in your forties, discuss this issue with your physician. If you are particularly fearful of breast cancer or have a number of breast cancer risk factors, you may indeed want to get a yearly test. To find a mammography center near you, call 800-4-CANCER.

Regular Breast Exams from a Health-Care Provider

All women should have their breasts examined by a doctor or nurse on a regular basis. How regular depends on your age: every three years if

21

you are between the ages of twenty and forty; every year if you are over forty, according to the American Cancer Society.

Regular Breast Self-Examination

Perform a monthly check of your breasts, at the same time in your cycle (see below).

Follow General Recommendations for Good Health

Quit smoking, exercise regularly, and don't drink in excess. Each of these lifestyle behaviors can reduce your risk for developing breast cancer.

Adopt a Cancer Prevention Diet

Eat a diet that is low in fat and protein and contains high quantities of disease-fighting antioxidants, beta carotene, soy, and omega-3 fatty acids. There are many foods—especially leafy greens and yellow and orange fruits and vegetables—that are known to lower your risk for breast cancer. The National Cancer Institute has found that women who eat at least five daily servings of fruits and vegetables have a lower rate of breast cancer than those who eat fewer than three. Conversely, the typical American diet, high in animal fat and protein, can increase your risk for disease. Substitute foods that contain omega-3 fatty acids (abundant in fish) and soy products, such as tofu, soy milk, and tempeh, which have been shown to protect women against breast cancer.

Consider Supplements and Alternative Prevention Strategies

Supplement your diet. If getting adequate quantities of fruits and vegetables is difficult for you, take a multivitamin supplement containing vitamins A, B, C, D, and E. The jury on beta-carotene supplements is still out; although foods rich in beta carotene are effective cancer fighters, some studies have shown that taking the nutrient in supplement form is not effective at preventing cancer. But research has demonstrated that other substances have tumor-fighting properties. One notable example: green tea, which is popular in Japanese restaurants.

The Breast Self-Exam

It's important to examine your breasts every month, preferably in the week following your period, since the breast changes throughout the menstrual cycle. The point of the breast self-exam is to become familiar

22

with the unique contours of your breasts. Once you have established this breast baseline, you will know if something has changed.

1. Start by visually scanning the breasts, looking for changes in the appearance, size, nipple color, and dimpling of skin.
2. Raise your arms and carefully look at your profile, repeating your observation on the other side.
3. Place your hands on your hips and press down hard while tensing the chest muscles. Repeat the visual assessment.
4. Lean forward and look for puckering of the skin, change in breast outline, and nipple retraction.
5. Lie on your back, putting your right hand behind your head. This makes the breast easier to palpate. If you have large breasts, place a pillow under the left shoulder. Examine your right breast with your left hand using these patterns of touch:

The Breast Self-Exam

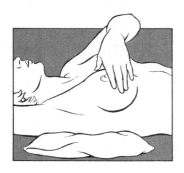
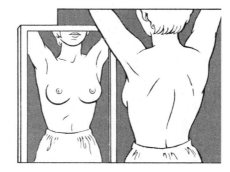
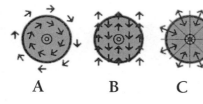
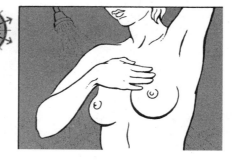

A. concentric circles
B. up-and-down motions
C. radial spoke motions

© American Cancer Society

All three patterns are necessary to thoroughly examine the breast. According to researchers at the University of Florida at Gainesville, using only concentric circles covers just 60 percent of the breast; the radial spoke technique covers only 45 percent of breast tissue. Make sure you also check the tissues in your armpit and along the top of the collarbone. Now repeat step five on the left breast.

Lumps Other than Cancer

Sometimes a lump is just a lump. If you find one during self-examination, chances are it is not dangerous. According to the *Mayo Clinic Health Letter,* several conditions can cause nonmalignant lumps, including *fibrocystic lumps,* which may feel ropy or granular. *Cysts* are fluid-filled sacs most often occurring in women ages thirty to fifty. These lumps often become tender right before menstruation. *Fibroadenomas* are benign tumors that feel solid, round, and rubbery. *Infection of a milk duct* can result in a reddened area that feels tender and lumpy. And lumps can be caused by a *bruise or blow* to the breast.

If a lump is discovered during your monthly self-check or through a mammogram, you likely will undergo a biopsy. According to the College of American Pathologists, if you have a lump that is benign, the pathologist will assign it to one of three categories based on its likelihood of presenting a later risk for breast cancer. If your biopsy indicates a condition such as fibrocystic breast disease, the biopsy will be characterized as presenting "no increased risk" for breast cancer. Your lump could also be designated as conferring a "slightly increased risk" (1.5 to 2 times) or a "moderately increased risk" (5 times). If you have lumps that fall into these latter categories, it is especially important to get mammograms on schedule, perform breast self-exams regularly, and take steps to prevent disease, as discussed earlier in this chapter.

Women need not suffer the consequences of neglect, fear, and ignorance regarding any aspect of their sexual and reproductive anatomy. Increasingly, women are putting aside the bodily shame that society has taught them makes women feminine in favor of regular screenings, open talks with their health-care providers, self-exams, and positive attitudes about their sexual health. You, too, can take this approach and enjoy the rewards of good health and fulfilling sex.

Breast Cancer Resources

Dr. Susan Love's Breast Book, by Susan Love, M.D. (Addison-Wesley, 1995).

Breast Cancer? Breast Health: The Wise Woman Way, by Susan S. Weed (Ashtree Publishing, 1996).

The Breast Book, by Miriam Stoppard, M.D. (Dorling Kinderslay Publishing, Inc., 1996).

Ordinary Life: A Memoir of Illness, by Kathlyn Conway (W. H. Freeman and Company, 1997).

National Breast Cancer Coalition
1707 L Street, NW, Suite 1060
Washington, DC 20036
202-296-7477

National Alliance of Breast Cancer Organizations
9 East 37th Street, 10th Floor
New York, NY 10016
800-719-9154

Susan G. Komen Breast Cancer Foundation
5005 LBJ Freeway, Suite 370
Dallas, TX 57244
800-Im-Aware (462-9273)

Y-Me National Breast Cancer Organization
212 West Van Buren Street
Chicago, IL 60607
312-986-8228 or 800-221-2141

3 | Feminine Rhythms

Menstruation is part of the cyclical processes that define women every day of their reproductive lives—not just the five days a month that they're having their periods. The following pages will help you understand what's normal, what's not, and how to address menstrual-related problems to stay in good health all month long.

This chapter also reconsiders the less-than-positive ideas many women have about menstruation. Seeing your period as part of a larger cycle—like the moon in shadow—is the place to start. It can increase your body awareness and may even help you shed negative attitudes about yourself and your body, which benefits your general sexual well-being.

A Menstrual Cycle Primer

While men produce sperm every day and for much of their lives, females are born with a finite number of egg cells needed for ovulation for their entire lifetimes. Of the million or so eggs available, some four hundred to five hundred will eventually be ovulated. At the time of her first period, a girl has started producing all the hormones involved in reproduction.

During the menstrual period (the time when a woman is actually bleeding), several egg follicles begin to mature inside the ovary, spurred by a hormone produced by the pituitary gland (the aptly named follicle-stimulating hormone). Day 1, the first day of the cycle, is the first day of bleeding. At this point, estrogen and progesterone levels, the key reproductive hormones, are low. Around Day 5, one egg follicle has grown largest, dwarfing the others. From Day 6 to Day 14 it continues to develop, releasing estrogen, which causes the lining in the uterus to thicken in preparation for the developing egg. Just prior to ovulation, estrogen levels drop a little and levels of the sex hormone androgen rise, which may enhance sexual feelings.

Ovulation happens when the egg breaks out of the follicle, leaves the ovary, and begins its journey through the fallopian tubes and into the uterus. As it grows, the egg begins to look yellow. Now referred to as the *corpus luteum* (or "yellow body"), it secretes increasing amounts of estrogen and progesterone. The progesterone rise triggers changes in the cervical mucus that influence the sperm's movement to the egg.

If the egg is fertilized by a sperm, pregnancy occurs. If pregnancy has not occurred by about Day 14, the cells of the corpus luteum begin to die and hormone levels drop. Without the hormones that thicken and enrich the uterine lining, it begins to shed as menstrual blood. Menstrual bleeding signals the brain to start the cycle all over again. A woman on the typical twenty-eight-day cycle starts bleeding on Day 29—Day 1 of the next menstrual cycle.

A note about what's normal: It's important to know that although 28 days is the length of the average cycle, cycles can vary significantly—from 21 to as many as 35 days. You are still normal even if you do not have a 28-day cycle.

I Got Rhythm: Charting Your Cycle

Whatever is normal for you, it's important to get to know your cycle. Becoming familiar with your own feminine rhythms can be extremely useful by giving you a baseline from which to observe physical changes that may indicate illness. You may also find that this cycle watching sensitizes you to hormone-related shifts. Many women feel more sexual or have greater energy around the time of ovulation. The simplest way to note your rhythm is to note the beginning of your cycle and keep a chart of symptoms that occur. Record the heaviness and texture of the flow, physical symptoms such as breast tenderness, and any emotional changes you may experience. You may identify patterns you suspected were there or find none where you assumed they existed.

Menstrual Myths and Blood Envy

Viewing menstruation through the lens of other societies can shed light on our own beliefs and traditions. Moreover, knowing that your culture plays a role in shaping your views about your period can help you change your negative menstruation views.

Myths about menstruation through history reveal the variety of human experience—from the sublime to the ridiculous. Women's cycles have influenced societies from the beginning of human history. Lunar markings found on prehistoric bone fragments show how early women marked their cycles and thus began to mark time. Women's periodic nature probably played a role in the development of counting and mathematics.

Menstrual blood was offered in ceremonies and considered sacred to the Celts, the ancient Egyptians, the Maoris, and the early Taoists. People of New Guinea, Australia, the Philippines, and Africa even developed blood-letting rituals for men, creating a kind of "men's menstruation."

In many societies, a girl's first period, or menarche, is a significant rite of passage. For example, newly menstruating Indian girls take ceremonial baths with their friends and rejoice at great feasts. The Manus of the South Pacific hold raucous splash parties in the lagoons, excluding men from the festivities. And Pygmy girls go into hiding at menarche with several young friends and an older female relative, later returning to a lengthy celebration.

In many Native American cultures, menstruation represents a time of self-growth and empowerment. "Within the Sioux culture, women were allowed time away from the group to renew. It was a time of personal reflection—to see where you've been, what parts of your life might need attention, and how to balance it out. It was time to be alone and not responsible for anything or busy with tasks," says Barbara Hanneloré, who teaches coming-of-age menstruation workshops in Ojai, California. "The Sioux believed menstruation is a woman's most receptive time and that it's easier to receive inspiration and vision if you are a little quieter."

Rituals have often been connected to women's monthly bleeding, and menstrual blood has been imbued with amazing powers. In various times menstrual blood was used to treat ailments from birthmarks to warts. It was thought to deflect evil spirits and even cure the plague.

More often, though, menstruation and menstruating women have been maligned. Many societies considered menstruation both mysterious and dangerous. According to *The Curse: A Cultural History of Menstruation* by Janice Delaney, Mary Jane Lupton, and Emily Toth, menstrual blood could make wine turn sour, metals rust, or crops fail.

Superstitions about menstrual blood are behind the myriad menstruation-related taboos of history and the common practice of banishing menstruating women from the larger group—sometimes to a hut or a lodge where they could not be seen by others. Menstruating women have often been thought to possess supernatural powers capable of endangering foods, a community, or a man's virility. Among the Zulus of Africa, for example, menstruating women are forbidden from eating milk curd or going near cows.

Not surprisingly, many cultures consider menstruation unclean. Lebanese Muslims prohibit menstruating women to have intercourse, enter cemeteries or mosques, or to be near a newborn child. Orthodox Jewish women take a purifying bath after their menses.

Our own culture frowns on menstruation. Although attitudes are beginning to change somewhat, secrecy and shame are still the norms. At best our periods are considered a nuisance, a monthly inconvenience that threatens our reputation as workers and our progress as equals in the working world. "Today's emphasis is on behaving normally during the menstrual period, and, be she housewife or career woman, today's woman is determined to prove she can do her job like a man even when she feels most like a woman," write the authors of *The Curse*.

Ignoring the defining feature of female biology defeats women by undermining their body image and self-esteem. As the culture teaches women to see their bodies as adversaries, many come to hate their own flesh. This body hatred serves only to erode their feelings of self-worth.

Conversely there is much to be gained by making peace with ourselves and by learning to work with our cycles, not against them. Acknowledging our own unique physical nature allows us to take greater pride in what we have to offer our partners, our children, our society, and ourselves.

Female Genital Mutilation

Among modern rites of passage, female genital mutilation (FGM) is one of the cruelest. FGM typically involves the partial or total removal of the clitoris and labia minora. In extreme cases, the insides of the labia majora are scraped, and the two sides of the vulva are stitched together or bound with thorns, leaving only a small hole for the passage of menstrual blood and urine. Formerly known as female circumcision, the practice is actually more akin to castration. Usually FGM is performed on girls between the ages of four and ten, often by older female relatives in unsanitary conditions and with no anesthesia.

According to the World Health Organization, between 85 and 114 million girls and women in the world are believed to have been so victimized. The practice, which has roots in ancient religious traditions, is regarded as a normal part of growing up in certain parts of Africa, the

Middle East, and, increasingly, in Islamic immigrant communities in the West. It is used to control women and to ensure their chastity before marriage.

The ritual itself is associated with extreme health consequences—shock, hemorrhage, infections, and even death. Many women who have been mutilated suffer lifelong health problems such as bladder and kidney disorders, chronic pain and infections, pregnancy complications, and loss of sexual sensitivity.

Several international health and human rights organizations, including the World Health Organization, are campaigning against the practice, and the issue received serious attention at the International Women's Conference in Beijing in 1995. FGM has also emerged as a controversial immigration issue in the United States and Canada. In recent years some women have sought asylum for themselves or their children to escape this harrowing tradition. Our courts are now grappling with the issue.

Menstrual Misfortunes

Fifty to 75 percent of women suffer from some physical or emotional distress during or near the time of their periods—from pain and nausea to mood swings, irritation, and bloating. Cramps are the most common complaint. Menstrual pain affects more than 30 million American women, accounting for some 600 million lost working days every year. According to the American College of Obstetricians and Gynecologists, more than 50 percent of women have some cramping for a day or two each month, while 10 to 15 percent have pain so severe that it interferes with their normal activities.

The Chemistry of Cramps

Most women feel cramps as an achiness or sense of pressure in the lower abdomen. The pain may extend to the hips, lower back, and even the inner thighs. Severe cramps can also trigger nausea, diarrhea, bloating, headache, or dizziness.

This type of cramping, occurring just before the menstrual period, is called primary dysmenorrhea. Common cramps typically start in adolescence and last into your twenties or until you have children. Primary dysmenorrhea is caused by the chemicals known as prostaglandins, which are produced in the uterine lining and released into the bloodstream when it's shed each cycle. These chemicals stimulate the contraction of the smooth muscle cells of the uterus. The more prostaglandins a woman produces, the greater her cramps. (Prostaglandins may also affect the cells in the intestinal tract, which explains why some women suffer from nausea and diarrhea during their monthly periods.)

Cures for Common Cramps

Drugs Now that doctors are wise to the causes of menstrual pain, they've developed a repertoire of pharmaceutical relief. Aspirin and acetaminophen are only so-so at taming cramps; ibuprofen-based drugs (Advil, Motrin), naproxen sodium (Aleve), and ketaprofen (Orudis) are better choices since they suppress the production of prostaglandins. Your best bet is to take a dose at the first sign of pain or even a day before you expect it to start.

If you have severe cramps, ask your health-care provider about the prescription version of naproxen sodium (Naprosyn, Anaprox) and other more powerful drugs, such as Ponstel, that reduce prostaglandin production. If you have killer cramps, your options include Toradol, a potent postoperative pain reliever.

The pill Oral contraceptives have the beneficial side effect of relieving menstrual pain.

Exercise Regular physical activity increases your body's mood-heightening endorphins and suppresses prostaglandin release.

Diet Meat, dairy products, and eggs are thought to contribute to the body's prostaglandin production. Fruits, vegetables, and whole grains—the gold standards of good nutrition—may help relieve your symptoms. Caffeine constricts blood flow, so cutting back may also help to reduce pain. Essential fatty acids, found in foods such as seeds, nuts, and salmon, may increase the production of anti-inflammatory prostaglandin hormones, thus easing cramping.

Alternative remedies Evening primrose oil, found in natural-food stores, also contains essential fatty acids that may help control pain. Black cohosh and black hawk bark may quell cramping by acting as

31

muscle relaxers—and white willow and feverfew are anti-inflammatories. A Chinese herb called Dang Gui or Dong-quai (which means "proper order") is often used to restore balance to the reproductive system and may reduce cramps.

Mysterious Mittelschmerz

If you've ever had a sudden, severe pain or cramp in your lower abdomen around the middle of your cycle, you may have experienced mittelschmertz, German for "middle pain." It happens when an ovary releases an egg. In some instances, the pain is so great it is confused with ectopic pregnancy or appendicitis.

Beyond Cramps

Sometimes a cramp is more than a cramp, signaling a more serious underlying problem. This type of painful period is called secondary dysmenorrhea. Here are the most common culprits:

Endometriosis

Symptoms

Very painful periods; heavy, irregular flow; chronic pain throughout the cycle, sometimes painful intercourse. In a third of sufferers there are no symptoms.

What It Is

The endometrium is a layer of tissue lining the uterus that is normally shed during the period. In some women, however, the endometrium attaches to body tissues outside the uterus, such as the ovaries, the fallopian tubes, or the vagina, and even the abdomen or intestines. During the menstrual period, this tissue (called implants or adhesions) bleeds just like the endometrium, but it has no place to go. Left unchecked, the bleeding can create scar tissue that spreads throughout the pelvic region, causing pain and potentially impairing your fertility. (Endometriosis is the primary cause of most cases of infertility in this country.) If your doctor suspects that you have endometriosis, she will probably schedule a procedure called laparoscopy, in which a tiny lighted scope is inserted through an incision in your belly button.

A MENSTRUAL FLOW CHART

Most women have some variability in their periods—from light flow to irregular periods. And usually there's an explanation, such as stress or fatigue. Usually these variations mean nothing more than a disruption in the body's normal rhythms. But sometimes the changes signal a more serious condition. If irregularities continue over several cycles, it's time to see a doctor. This chart outlines some typical problems and their possible causes, but only a health-care provider can properly diagnose and treat your condition.

Condition: Light Bleeding/Short Periods

Possible Causes

Hormonal contraceptives, menopause, stress, drugs for psychological disorders, early pregnancy, sexually transmitted diseases (STD).

Condition: Irregular Periods

Possible Causes

Polycystic ovary syndrome (an imbalance of hormones that causes long gaps between periods), weight loss or gain, thyroid problems, travel across time zones or other disruptions to circadian rhythms, ectopic pregnancy (when the embryo implants outside the uterus), stress.

Condition: Heavy Bleeding/Long Periods

Possible Causes

Fibroid tumors, failure to ovulate due to hormone problems, endometriosis, miscarriage, IUD use.

Condition: Breakthrough Bleeding

Possible Causes

Ectopic pregnancy, change in oral contraceptive dose or a missed dose, uterine fibroids or polyps, infection triggered by an IUD, cancer of the cervix or uterus (especially if bleeding occurs after intercourse or after using tampons), ovarian cysts, STDs (especially chlamydia and gonorrhea).

Condition: Amenorrhea (lack of periods)

Possible Causes

Pregnancy, menopause, excessive exercise, presence of eating disorder, stress, polycystic ovary syndrome, drugs for certain psychological problems.

What to Do

Pregnancy used to be the only "cure" for endometriosis, aside from hysterectomy. And while becoming pregnant may temporarily reduce the symptoms, the problem often returns. Your provider may prescribe hormonal treatments that stop menstruation, curbing the development of the misplaced tissue. GnRH analogs (Lupron, Suprefact, Synarel, and Zoladex) are the most effective treatments, though, as is true with all drugs used to treat endometriosis, they have significant side effects. If your doctor finds endometrial adhesions during laparoscopy, she may be able to remove them with a laser during the procedure. But if the tissue is extensive, more surgery may be necessary. In the most extreme cases, hysterectomy may be required.

Fibroid Tumors

Symptoms

Heavy bleeding, pain, swollen abdomen, painful intercourse; sometimes no symptoms.

What It Is

A fibroid is a tumor, usually benign, that develops inside the uterus, within the uterine wall. Fibroids often occur in women between the ages of thirty and fifty, and they are more common in black women, although researchers don't know why. One theory is that black women are more likely to carry a gene, as yet unidentified, that influences the development of fibroids. One in four women will be diagnosed with fibroid tumors during her reproductive years. Though the cause of fibroids is unknown, many researchers believe the tumors are related to high levels of estrogen. Fibroids may in fact get larger during early pregnancy, when levels of the hormone are high, and they tend to disappear after menopause, when estrogen is in decline. Fibroids can often be felt during a pelvic exam or diagnosed with ultrasound or surgery.

What to Do

Most women do not require treatment, but your provider may recommend surgery to remove the fibroids or the uterus if there is excessive bleeding, sudden enlargement of the fibroid, or unbearable pain. A hysterectomy is sometimes required. Doctors may also prescribe a class of drugs called GnRH agonists, which temporarily suppress estrogen production. But menopausal symptoms may develop as a side effect to these drugs.

Ovarian Cysts

Symptoms

Fullness or pain in the lower abdomen, pain during intercourse.

What It Is

A cyst is a fluid-filled sac that forms inside the ovary during ovulation. An ovarian cyst is usually harmless unless it becomes very large.

What to Do

Often cysts disappear on their own. Your health-care provider will probably wait two or three months to see if it goes away. Sometimes birth control pills are prescribed to help shrink a cyst. Oral contraceptives prevent ovulation and also help block the development of new cysts. (Indeed, women on birth control pills rarely get ovarian cysts.) When cysts are very large or cause severe pain, they must be surgically removed. If you have ever experienced a sudden, intense pain on one side that occurred midcycle and disappeared within twenty-four hours, you may have had a cyst that ruptured.

Pelvic Inflammatory Disease (PID)

Symptoms

A dull ache and tenderness in the abdomen, sometimes vaginal discharge or fever, pain during pelvic exam; sometimes no symptoms.

What It Is

An infection often caused by the sexually transmitted diseases gonorrhea or chlamydia or associated with the insertion of an IUD. PID can lead to infertility and a greater risk for ectopic pregnancy. It is diagnosed through blood tests, ultrasound, or laparoscopy.

What to Do

The treatment is a course of antibiotics. Since PID can recur and is linked with sexually transmitted diseases, it's important to practice safe sex. Barrier methods, such as condoms, diaphragms, and spermicides, provide greater protection against PID because they block the cervix. Oral contraceptives may hinder the movement of bacteria through the reproductive tract. Women with more than one sexual partner should not use IUDs because they may promote infection, however.

Hysterectomy Alert

Doctors perform more than 500,000 hysterectomies each year in the United States, making them one of the most frequently performed surgeries. According to the National Center for Health Statistics, one in three women in the United States has had a hysterectomy by the age of sixty.

Hysterectomies are performed to prevent the spread of cancer in the reproductive system, and they are also frequently performed for abnormal bleeding, fibroid tumors, endometriosis, and uterine prolapse. But many of these hysterectomies may be unnecessary: Only 10 percent are performed for cancer; the other 90 percent are for nonmalignant conditions for which there may be alternatives. A study conducted by the Rand Corporation in 1993 found that surgery was appropriate only in 58 percent of cases. It was inappropriate in 16 percent of cases and questionable in 25 percent.

Although a hysterectomy can free a woman of pelvic pain, excessive bleeding, depression, and urinary tract problems, it can also inflict a new array of symptoms, including some of these same complaints. The traditional hysterectomy procedure often involves the removal of the ovaries along with the uterus, a procedure called bilateral oophorectomy, which can plunge a woman into premature menopause. The abrupt halt to the hormones that the ovaries produce can seriously affect her quality of life. In many cases the cervix is removed along with the uterus, which tends to shorten the vagina. This can adversely affect a woman's sexual experience. Women who undergo hysterectomies are also often subject to menopausal symptoms—from lagging sex drive to vaginal dryness.

Even if a woman is near menopause, removing her ovaries comes at a significant price. According to Donna Shoupe, M.D., a professor of obstetrics and gynecology at the University of Southern California School of Medicine in Los Angeles, the ovaries continue to produce helpful hormones well after menopause. All postmenopausal ovaries make some estrogen, protecting women against a host of ills, including heart disease, osteoporosis, and even declines in brain function. Ovaries also produce some 60 percent of the testosterone that's produced before a woman reaches menopause. "Testosterone is by itself wonderful for bones," Shoupe says. "It also enhances muscle strength and confers a sense of well-being." Testosterone also plays a role in maintaining libido.

Many women are unaware of the possible changes that can occur with the surgery. Ask your doctor to spell out the risks and consequences of hysterectomy, and consider getting a second opinion if the surgery is recommended.

The Alternatives

There are several alternative treatments for hysterectomies. For example, *myomectomy* is a surgical removal of fibroid tumors that spares the uterus. (Although often associated with significant complications, it may be a good option when a patient wants to preserve the right to have children.) Two other surgical procedures can often relieve the symptoms of endometriosis. They are *laparoscopy,* an outpatient procedure involving a thin scope that's inserted through a small incision in the belly button, and *laparotomy,* a more extensive surgery performed through small cuts in the abdomen. Bleeding problems can often be alleviated with hormonal treatments or dilatation and curettage (D&C)—scraping the endometrium, or uterine lining.

A procedure called *endometrial ablation* removes the uterine lining but leaves the uterus intact. This procedure has emerged in recent years as a promising new treatment for excessive bleeding due to a newly designed surgical instrument that makes it a smoother surgery. Other researchers are conducting trials of *balloon ablation,* a variation on this method inspired by balloon angioplasty. With *uterine artery embolization,* surgeons cut off the blood supply to fibroids so they can't grow.

Even if the uterus is surgically removed, however, there are important reasons to consider—and request—that the ovaries remain intact.

"When would a man consider having his testicles removed and taking a testosterone pill every day for the rest of his life?" asks Shoupe. "It's the same thing with the ovaries. Why take out a functioning organ when we now know the benefits they provide transitionally into menopause and even into late menopause?"

Many doctors are unaware of the new medical procedures that could help a woman avoid hysterectomies and oopherectomies. "The surgery techniques are better today. Doctors used to remove everything because they didn't want to take the risks of having to go back in later if the need arose. With laparoscopic surgical techniques, the risk-benefit balance has changed. And until recently, we didn't know how valuable these hormones are. Doctors need to catch up on and provide women with the information to make realistic judgments," Shoupe says. Similar arguments can be made about saving the cervix. According to Shoupe, preserving the cervix actually simplifies the surgical procedure.

If your doctor is unaware of alternatives to hysterectomy or is unwilling to consider a cervix or ovary-sparing hysterectomy, get a second opinion—or a new doctor.

The Menace of PMS

Technically, a diagnosis of PMS—premenstrual syndrome—means that a woman experiences five or more PMS-related symptoms. The list includes acne, anxiety, fatigue, weight gain, tension, insomnia, irritability, nausea, depression, bloating, breast tenderness, constipation, food cravings, forgetfulness, and a host of other problems.

Premenstrual Dysphoric Disorder (PMDD) is a more serious psychiatric disorder that markedly impairs a woman's ability to work or interact with others. Women with PMDD have at least five of eleven specific symptoms: depression, anxiety or tension, mood swings, anger or irritability, decreased sexual desire, difficulty in concentrating, lethargy, appetite changes or food cravings, sleep problems, a feeling of being "out of control," and physical symptoms, such as headaches, muscle pain, breast tenderness, and weight gain.

Most of us manage the annoying days before our periods with pain killers and a little patience. For some women, however, bloating, mood swings, irritability, depression, tension, or headaches rock the very roots of life. So while most women's premenstrual problems put a damper on the day, women with PMS and PMDD have trouble simply getting through it.

With all the possible means of distress, it's not surprising that there is no universally accepted criteria for diagnosing PMS. So doctors focus on two things when making a diagnosis: the severity of symptoms and their occurrence. To be considered menstrual related, the symptoms must occur only during the luteal phase of the cycle, which begins with ovulation (around Day 12 to 16) and continues until the start of the next menstrual period. If symptoms occur at other times in the cycle, PMS is not the problem.

Experts estimate that 20 to 25 percent of women have no symptoms prior to their periods. Some 75 to 80 percent have a at least some symptoms,with 2 to 3 percent exhibiting bona fide PMS. A small number—3 to 5 percent of normally cycling women—have PMDD.

Doctors don't know why some women have premenstrual problems and others sail through the premenstrual phase symptom free. According to Jean Endicott, Ph.D., director of the Premenstrual Evaluation Unit of the Columbia-Presbyterian Medical Center in New York City, the prevailing theory is that the problem lies in widely fluctuating levels of serotonin, one of the body's mood-regulating hormones.

Serotonin is probably just a piece of the puzzle. Research has also suggested that the ratio of estrogen to progesterone during the cycle may play a role. And new data hints that receptors for these hormones may malfunction in women with PMS.

Because diagnosis can be difficult, your doctor or health-care provider will probably ask you to keep a daily symptom diary for at least two menstrual cycles, charting the three to five worst symptoms. This diary process helps to determine whether symptoms are linked to the menstrual cycle. Your provider will also rule out other psychiatric disorders.

Keeping the diary can also help you monitor your moods so you know when to expect the worst cycle-related symptoms. If you expect PMS, you can reschedule important meetings, make sleep a priority, or treat yourself well. In fact, simply getting a diagnosis of PMS represents a huge relief to some women: It says their problem has a biological basis and that they aren't mentally ill.

Fortunately, medicine has been expanding its repertoire of drug treatments for women with debilitating premenstrual symptoms. And many seek relief from simple dietary changes and alternative therapies. Here are some of the currently used therapies that may be of use to you if you experience PMS:

Diet

- Research shows that eating carbohydrate-rich, low-fat foods may affect serotonin levels and lesson mood symptoms and other PMS woes. It's also good to eat multiple small meals.
- Essential fatty acids, contained in foods like salmon, seeds, and soybeans, or in evening primrose oil, can be helpful in reducing pain.
- Caffeine appears to worsen symptoms, so try to cut back. (Drink half-caffeinated, half-decaffeinated beverages for a week, then gradually wean yourself completely.)
- Calcium-rich foods help to cut down on water retention.
- Contrary to common thought, reducing your salt intake may not help ease bloating, according to a 1996 study conducted by the National Institutes of Health. Women who were menstruating reduced their salt intake but experienced no reduction in swelling and breast tenderness.

Vitamins

Although medical evidence is mixed, vitamins, particularly vitamin B_6, help some women live with PMS. Many doctors recommend a daily multivitamin and B_6 (50 milligrams daily). Don't exceed 150 milligrams daily of B_6 since high levels of the vitamin can be toxic.

Exercise

Regular physical activity helps ease depression and cramping. Aerobic exercise unleashes mood-elevating endorphins and boosts serotonin, both of which may counteract depressive tendencies.

Drugs

- Recently doctors have turned to a class of drugs known as selective serotonin reuptake inhibitors, or SSRIs, for the treatment of serious premenstrual symptoms. Prozac, Paxil, and Zoloft are three of the SSRIs that help regulate serotonin and thus help reduce mood-related symptoms. In drug trials, women on these medications felt more energetic, content, and in control during their periods. Xanax, a popular antianxiety medication, is somewhat less effective.
- Progesterone is another commonly prescribed drug therapy, but its research record is mixed.
- For heavy-duty cases, doctors may suggest GnRH agonists to suppress the production of estrogen and progesterone. However, the drugs also stop menstruation, triggering a kind of temporary menopause. Because these drugs enhance the risk for osteoporosis, they are only used for a few months at a time.

All of these drugs have side effects. Ask your doctor to spell out the possible problems you may encounter before you try them.

Alternative Therapies

- Several research studies have suggested that women with PMS may experience relief through traditional Chinese medicine. Acupuncture—the ancient practice of applying needles to specific points in the body to affect positive changes—is one part of a four-pronged strategy involving exercise, certain herbs (in particular, the herb known as Dang Gui or Dong-quai), and a balanced diet that emphasizes grains, vegetables, and fruits. In general the diet calls for the following ratio of foods: 50 percent grains, 20 percent vegetables, 10 percent fruits, 10 percent protein, 5 percent legumes, and less than 5 percent oils, sweets, and fats.

- Reflexology is an alternative treatment based on the notion that applying pressure to points on the feet and hands helps heal other places in the body. In a study published in *Obstetrics and Gynecology* in 1994, women had a 46 percent reduction in PMS symptoms after using reflexology.

- Women may find help for emotional and physical distress in relaxation techniques such as yoga, meditation, and biofeedback.

- Many herbs are thought to be helpful in treating PMS symptoms. Valerian root, hops, and passion flower act as sedatives to calm the nervous system and promote sleep. Parsley, dandelion, and sarsaparilla appear to decrease bloating and water retention. Black cohosh, black hawk, and white willow bark may be useful against pain. Don't mix herbs with drugs, however, and let your doctor know that you are taking herbs.

A New View of Menstruation: Don't Cramp My Style

When it comes to coping with painful periods and PMS, negative societal attitudes toward menstruation are no help. In the wry, thought-provoking essay "If Men Could Menstruate," feminist Gloria Steinem muses that were biological roles reversed, "menstruation would become an enviable, boastworthy event: Men would brag about how long and how much. Young boys would talk about it as the envied beginning of manhood. . . . Sanitary supplies would be federally funded and free."

Janice Delaney, Mary Jane Tupton, and Emily Toth, authors of *The Curse: A Cultural History of Menstruation,* had a similar brainstorm one day. The upshot: a list of ten "symptoms" of menstruation that don't usually come up when women talk about their periods. The list included "creativity," "increased sexual desire," and "intense concentration"—not so far-fetched. But other items—"euphoria," "high spirits" and, especially, "revolutionary zeal"—required a playful stretch of the imagination.

"It started out as a consciousness-raising joke. No one looks for the positive aspects of menstruation. Our culture's focus is on the negativity," says Joan C. Chrisler, Ph.D., a professor of psychology at Connecticut College in New London, who decided to actually use the questionnaire, titled, "Menstrual Joy," in a study with a group of college students. Her

41

motive: to see whether women have any favorable menstrual symptoms and whether the test itself might spur an attitude adjustment. In fact, Chrisler suspected that researchers reinforce negative attitudes toward menstruation by assuming the worst. (One of the standard tests for determining attitudes toward menstruation is even called the Menstrual *Distress* Questionnaire.)

What did she find? Two-thirds of the women reported that they had never considered menstruation to be a positive event, and one in three thought they would view their periods differently in the future as a result of participating in the study. Clearly the way menstruation is portrayed to women influences their experience of it.

As far as actual symptoms, a number of women reported positive changes when menstruating, particularly increased sexual desire, feelings of affection, and improved self-confidence. According to Chrisler, affection and libido may fluctuate with hormonal shifts. And anecdotal reports of enhanced creativity pop up frequently in the journals of famous women, though there is scant data to back it up.

In several other studies, women have noted additional positive shifts, courtesy of their monthly period—heightened sensitivity to their environment and vividly revealing dreams, among them. A University of Texas study found that women who had PMS demonstrated greater abilities of perception at certain times in the cycle, an effect that researchers chalked up to fluctuating levels of the neurotransmitter serotonin.

Some maverick scientists are also shedding new light on the process, offering new theories that have the power to change menstruation's much maligned reputation. Margie Profet, an evolutionary biologist and MacArthur Fellowship (the "genius grant") winner, believes that menstruation's role is to rid a woman's body of pathogens that hitchhike on sperm into the female reproductive tract during intercourse. According to her theory, uterine shedding is a self-cleaning mechanism designed to keep toxins from infecting a woman's reproductive organs.

The concept may be beneficial to women. As Profet told *Omni* magazine: "One way my theory may help is that many men hold disdainful attitudes toward menstruation and of women having to go through this bizarre, girly thing. Maybe now, they'll have a little more respect for it."

A little respect wouldn't hurt women, either. Developing a healthy sexual self-awareness means tuning into all the changes your body experiences during your cycle. If you expect something good, you might find it. But if you are convinced otherwise, you may never notice anything positive.

The "Menstrual Joy" Questionnaire

During your next period, note whether and when these symptoms occur:

High spirits
Increased sexual desire
Vibrant activity
Revolutionary zeal
Intense concentration
Feelings of affection
Self-confidence
Sense of euphoria
Creativity
Feelings of power

Blood Sisters: The Menstruation Movement

"Our culture offers two choices: We can either pretend that menstruation is not happening or we can resent it," says Barbara Hanneloré, who teaches workshops on menstruation in Ojai, California. She and other like-minded women hope to change women's perceptions about their periods by teaching women and girls to value their cycles as a treasured facet of their femininity and by reclaiming lost traditions that celebrate menstrual cycling.

One of the menstruation movement's most prominent figures is Tamara Slayton, director of the Menstrual Health Foundation in Sebastopol, California, who pioneered the idea of coming-of-age workshops for girls. At her Camp Fertility workshops, newly menstruating girls learn about the mysteries of their changing bodies and play games that celebrate their new status, such as building fertility goddesses out of the sand. The weekends close with a celebration in which the girls are crowned "queens of fertility" by their proud families.

Hanneloré, offering similar workshops, hopes to spare girls from the silence, shame, and secrecy that marked many of their mothers' own comings of age. Girls learn to chart their periods in a first stab at fertility awareness, and their mothers honor them with poems at a postworkshop celebration. "I try to bring as much beauty and significance to the event as I can. We hope they learn a healthy way of self-care that can benefit them their whole lives," Hanneloré says.

Even if you began menstruating long ago, however, advocates of men-

GO WITH THE FLOW

While you may not wish to go so far as to participate in an organized cycle-celebrating ritual, honoring your identity as a woman can be important to your self-esteem and body image. Hanneloré suggests creating your own personal ritual, such as lighting a candle or wearing a special bracelet during your period. Use the time to be quiet and creative.

"I draw a red line on my calendar a month ahead of time," Hanneloré says. "That way I don't fill in those days with frantic activity. When the time arrives, I have a choice. I find that when I have my period, I don't want to interact too much with others or follow a schedule." Even if you have no control over your work schedule, you can arrange other activities around your period and make time to care for yourself. Hire a baby-sitter, for instance, or sleep in on the weekend.

strual awareness believe you can change your period perspective. Much of their work is aimed at women who missed being honored for being women. Learning to respect their own bodily processes means challenging deeply ingrained negative ideas about their bodies and themselves. Making the effort offers physical as well as psychological rewards, Hanneloré says—including easing premenstrual symptoms.

"Simply acknowledging that you may need time alone can do wonders," she says. "I encourage women to observe with curiosity and care what their bodies are telling them. When we're running around trying to ignore the fact that we would rather be withdrawing a little from our busy lives, we can enhance our discontent."

Some women now organize coming-of-age ceremonies for themselves or groups of friends. Hanneloré's coming-of-age cohorts sat around a fire and told stories about their first menstrual periods, imagined the beginnings they would like to have had, exchanged gifts, and dyed scarves red to signify menstrual blood. At the end of the celebration, they wrapped themselves in the scarves, danced, and blessed themselves.

For information on Slayton's programs including correspondence courses, contact Womankind, Products, Programs, and Publications for Loving Your Cycle, P.O. Box 1775, Sebastopol, California 95473; 707-522-8662; Web site: http://www.ensemble.com/womankind.

Creating a Positive Rite of Passage

How parents, relatives, and friends treat a girl's menarche shapes her views about menstruation, her body, and sex for a lifetime. When families ignore a girl's first period, she understands that menstruation is shameful and embarrassing. But families can communicate that menstruation is a positive event. A father's affirmation and respect is particularly important to a girl's developing self-esteem.

In her research, Joan Chrisler, Ph.D., asked women to describe their memories of menarche. In the stories that stood out, the women had been honored with symbolic gestures. "Some fathers gave their daughters a red rose," Chrisler says. "Nothing was said, but the symbolism was very important to them." Parents can offer their daughters a glass of red wine at dinner, which also acknowledges their new adult status. Or female relatives—mothers, grandmothers, or aunts—can take girls out to a special lunch. "We need to do something," says Chrisler, "to make this seem like a rite of passage—like a positive thing."

Period Pieces: New Menstrual Wares

Women who question the menstruation myths in our culture also question the use of disposable menstruation products, especially tampons, which help women conceal the fact that they're menstruating.

A thriving alternative menstrual industry seeks to fill the demand. Several companies now peddle so-called moon pads or wraps, washable cotton pads in pretty flannels, and sea sponges designed to "catch the flow."

Such products also appeal to the environmentally conscious, since they are designed to be reused and not burden landfills. Indeed, menstruation generates big business—and a lot of waste. Some 11.3 billion sanitary pads were landfilled or incinerated in 1990. The average American woman (menstruating from twelve to forty-two, five days a month, and using five tampons per day) theoretically uses nearly twelve thousand tampons during her reproductive lifetime.

Tampon manufacturers are also responding to rising health and environmental concerns about conventional tampons that are bleached with chlorine. Although the effects of bleached tampons on women's health has not been fully explored, there's evidence that repeated exposure to dioxin may present some reproductive health risks. Dioxin residues have been found on major tampon brands. No one knows how much dioxin a woman may be exposed to without suffering harm. But a number of tampon manufacturers now market unbleached, all-cotton tampons.

For information on alternative menstrual pads and tampons, contact:

- Womankind, Products, Programs, and Publications for Loving Your Cycle, P.O. Box 1775, Sebastopol, CA 95473; 707-522-8662; Web site: http://www.ensemble.com/womankind.
- Glad Rags, P.O. Box 12751, Portland, OR 97212; 800-799-4523 (cotton menstrual pads).
- Natural Concepts, Lotus Trading Company, 4128½ California Avenue, SW, Suite 168, Seattle, WA 98116; 206-932-7191, 888-515-5262 (pads, accessories, and kits).
- The Keeper, P.O. Box 20023, Cincinnati, OH 45220 (a rubber device that works like a diaphragm to catch menstrual blood).
- The Sea Sponge, Sea Sponges, Medea Books, 849 Almar Avenue, Suite C-285, Santa Cruz, CA 95060; 800-41-MEDEA.
- Women's Choice, 3415 Juriet Road, RR#3 Ladysmith, BC, V0R 2E0, Canada; 205-772-7013, fax: 250-722-7019.

A basement in a suburban Maryland ranch house is the last place you'd expect to find the world's only museum devoted to menstruation. But there's an even bigger surprise: The Museum of Menstruation was created by a man.

Harry Finley, a graphic designer, is the first to admit his lack of firsthand knowledge. "I'm just a guy," he says, "an outsider." What he lacks in X chromosomes, however, Finley makes up for with enthusiasm for his subject. The collection contains more than a thousand items of menstruation memorabilia—from turn-of-the-century Kotex ads to ecologically correct menstrual products. Together they offer a revealing glimpse of society's repressive attitudes about sex and the role of advertising in maintaining the menstruation taboo.

Open to the public in 1994, the museum features feminine hygiene advertisements from the United States, Japan, Germany, and Swe-

- Feminine Options, Thirtieth Street, Ridgeland, WI 54763; 715-455-1652 (a line of "menstrual lingerie"—washable holders and liners).

For chlorine-free paper tampons and pads:

- Natracare, 191 University Boulevard, Suite 219, Denver, CO 80206.
- Terra Femme (chlorine-free tampons), Bio Business International Inc., 78 Hallam Street, Toronto, ON, Canada M6H 1W8; 416-539-8548, fax: 416-539-9784.
- Seventh Generation, Colchester, VT 05446-1672; 800-456-1177.
- Today's Choice, 500 American Way, King of Prussia, PA 19406; 800-262-0042.
- Women and Environments Education and Development (WEED), 736 Bathurst Street, Toronto, Canada ON M5S 2R4, 416-516-2600; fax: 416-531-6214.

New Dry Ideas

It's been awhile since we've witnessed any revolutionary trends in feminine protection (unless you count the wings that have sprouted on some brands of minipads). After all, the last real innovation—the tampon—was introduced way back in 1936.

But the options for menstruating women have recently expanded, thanks to two new products. The first is called Instead. Made of a soft, flexible plastic, Instead is a disposable cup that is worn internally to trap the menstrual flow (unlike the Keeper, which is intended to be reused). The manufacturers claim the diaphragmlike device creates a snug seal and can be safely left in place for up to twelve hours—even during sexual intercourse. (Instead is not a contraceptive and will not guard against pregnancy or sexually transmitted diseases.) Available in drugstores, Instead can also be ordered by mail (888-367-9636). A box of six cups costs about $2; fourteen cups for about $5.

In Sync Miniforms are small (two-and-one-half-inch) rolls that are actually held in place by the vaginal lips, or labia. They are designed to be used as a backup to tampons and pads on heavy flow days and by themselves on light days. They can also be worn to absorb vaginal creams (if or when you're being treated for a yeast infection), slight urine leakage, and vaginal discharge. To order the Miniform, call 800-700-8716.

Tampons and Toxic Shock Syndrome

If you were menstruating in 1979 and 1980, no doubt you can recall the toxic shock syndrome (TSS) scare. This rare but dangerous disease, caused by a *Staphylococcus* bacteria, struck some eight hundred women, most of whom were using superabsorbent synthetic tampons—particularly a brand called Rely. Such tampons were capable of absorbing more moisture than was actually in the vagina. Left in place for several hours, the tampons were sometimes hard to remove, and they left residues of the synthetic materials and small lacerations in the vaginal walls, promoting the growth of the unhealthy bacteria.

Fortunately the tampons implicated in the TSS scare cannot be found on drugstore shelves today, and doctors and scientists have learned a lot about the "bug" that causes TSS. While the incidence of TSS has dropped and the disease is now extremely rare, one in a hundred thousand women still gets menstruation-related TSS each year, according to the Centers for Disease Control. (Women who use a diaphragm or cervical cap for birth control also have a slightly increased risk for toxic shock.)

Though small, these risks are real because the vaginal environment offers an ideal breeding ground for the TSS bacteria under the right conditions. Women under thirty—and particularly women ages fifteen to nineteen—are more susceptible to the disease. Your chances of contracting TSS decrease if you use appropriate tampons for your needs (super on heavy flow days, regular on lighter ones). Use them intermittently, alternating with pads throughout the period. Doctors recommend using pads on light flow days and refraining from wearing tampons overnight.

The FDA currently recommends changing tampons every six to eight hours, but some experts recommend changing more frequently. Just to compound confusion, some health experts caution that it's possible to change tampons *too* frequently: If you remove a tampon before it has absorbed much fluid, say, after two or three hours, you can irritate the vaginal walls, possibly even promoting infection. Many physicians now advise women to change tampons every four hours.

Consider using an all-cotton tampon. (*See "Period Pieces," page 45.*) A 1994 study by researchers at the Tisch Hospital/New York University Medical Center found that all-cotton tampons produce none of the TSS bacteria. Conversely, most major brands that contain synthetic materials *increase* the production of the bacteria—at least under laboratory conditions.

den—many of them guilty of promoting secrecy and shame. The museum also holds art by and about menstruation and information on biological aspects of our monthly periods.

According to Finley, the most popular item in the collection is part of an art project created by a graduate student at the University of Iowa. The artist, Teresa Konechne, filled up six hundred sanitary napkin boxes (like those you find on airplanes) with stories she'd collected from women about their first periods. Fifteen of these boxes now reside on Finley's rec-room wall. "Women warm up to these right away. It seems to foster a sense of community among them," he says, summing up the museum's raison d'etre.

Fittingly, the museum is only open at certain times of the month—by appointment. For more information, write the Museum of Menstruation, or MUM, Box 2398, Landover, MD 20784-2398; 301-459-4450, or visit MUM's Web site: http://www.mum.org.

Remove your tampon and contact a doctor or hospital if you develop any of these symptoms during your period:

- high fever (at least 102 degrees)
- nausea
- a diffuse red rash, especially on the torso (looks like raspberries or sunburn)
- rapidly falling blood pressure, dizziness
- diarrhea
- muscle aches
- peeling skin

Resources

SPOT, the Tampon Health Web site:
http://www.critpath.org/~tracy/spot.html

Endometriosis Association
8585 N. Seventy-Sixth Place
Milwaukee, WI 53223
800-992-3636
A self-help organization for sufferers.

Endometriosis Treatment Program
St. Charles Medical Center
2500 N.E. Neff Road
Bend, OR 97701
800-446-2177, ext. 6904

HERS Foundation
(Hysterectomy Educational Resources and Services)
422 Bryn Mawr Avenue
Bala Cynwyd, PA 19004
610-667-7757; fax: 610-667-8096

4 Contraceptive Consciousness

Perfect Contraception?

Nearly half of unintended pregnancies happen to women *using* birth control.

If you find this fact alarming, it's time for a reality check about contraception. The stated effectiveness of contraceptive products and devices is based on what is called "perfect use." In the real world, people tend to lower these pristine research figures significantly. Indeed, experts agree that it's women and their partners who are failing their methods—not the other way around. For instance, a study from the University of North Carolina at Chapel Hill found that 47 percent of women on oral contraceptives miss a pill at least once a month, and 22 percent miss two or more, dramatically increasing their odds of getting pregnant.

Birth control can be messy, inconvenient, and generally less than perfect. It's no wonder people slip up, or simply give up, on their contraception.

But there's more to the story than user failure. The radical changes in health care over the last decade have diminished a woman's opportunities to learn the facts about birth control from her health-care provider. For the increasing numbers of women in managed-care programs, time with a doctor is brief and getting briefer. The details of contraception take time.

Even if you *think* you are utilizing your birth control method correctly and consistently—the two commandments of contraceptive usage—there may be some facts about your chosen method that you don't know, facts that could maximize its effectiveness in preventing pregnancy and nudge you a tad closer to perfect use. The more you know about your chosen method, the better it can work for you.

Boosting your contraceptive confidence has other attractive benefits, such as letting you relax and enjoy the pleasures of sex. You can forget about that if you're wondering whether your diaphragm is in the right position or trying to decide if the condoms in your nightstand are still effective. It's easy to see why one of the best things you can do for your love life is to get better acquainted with your birth control.

Birth Control: A Primer

In this section, you'll find detailed descriptions of the popular methods of birth control if you're in the market for a new method or simply want to find out more about your current method. *The Basics* provides an overview: an explanation of how each method works, failure rates for perfect and typical use, and the approximate cost. The *Ideal User* section is intended to share some common characteristics of the methods' users. A list of method *Pros* and *Cons* follows.

Whatever a method's limitations, its effectiveness can almost always be improved. It's a good idea to carefully read the instructions that come with your birth control product or device. The *Tips for Smart Sex* for each contraceptive method provide additional hints to help reduce your worry. *The Feel-Good Factor* offers information about the contraceptive method and sexual pleasure.

Deciding which contraception to use is a complex decision, involving your health, age, personality, and personal preferences. No one method is right for everyone. Women must weigh both the risks and benefits of the available methods in concert with their health-care providers.

Lunatic Fringe Sperm *(and Other Amazing Sperm Facts)*

They're fast, aggressive, and will stop at nothing to reach their goal. Is your contraception up to the sperm challenge?

- The average sperm's survival is about three to four days in the female genital tract. But since there are 300 million sperm in a normal ejaculate, some of them—one sexual health expert dubs them "lunatic fringe sperm"—can survive in the genital tract up to seven days.
- If every sperm in the normal ejaculate—about one teaspoon—were able to fertilize an egg, any one man could populate all of North America on a single occasion.
- Sperm, with an average swimming speed of three millimeters per minute, reach the upper genital tract in less than three to five minutes and into the fallopian tubes on the order of ten minutes.
- Scientists have identified superaggressive "kamikaze sperm" that block the passage of or even kill competing sperm.

> ### A Sexist Sperm Joke
>
> Question: *Why does it take so many sperm to fertilize an egg?*
> Answer: *Because none of them will stop and ask for directions.*

Condoms and Spermicide

The Basics

The condom is the only contraceptive method that protects against both pregnancy and STDs. Usually made of latex rubber, condoms are rolled onto an erect penis before any contact with the genitals because sperm can be found in the "pre-ejaculate"—the clear fluid that emerges in the early stages of sexual arousal. (New polyurethane condoms can be used by people who are allergic to latex.) Some condoms (including those made with lambskin) do not protect against STDs, but condoms that do will state it on the packaging. Using a spermicide—over-the-counter creams, foams, and jellies that kill sperm—increases a condom's effectiveness significantly. The active ingredient in many spermicides is nonoxynol-9, which may be somewhat effective against HIV, the virus that causes AIDS.

Failure rate: 3 percent perfect use, 12 percent typical use.

Cost: 50¢ or less (spermicide: 25¢ per use).

Ideal User

The condom is best for women and their partner(s) who want the birth control method with the one-two punch: contraception *and* disease protection. Users enjoy the lack of health risks or side effects, and ideally possess the self-control, assertiveness, and discipline to use it with each act of intercourse.

Pros

- Requires no medical exam or prescription.
- Inexpensive to use.
- Prevents STDs, including AIDS.
- Helps some men delay ejaculation.

Cons

- The interruption of foreplay is a drawback for some people.
- Requires cooperation from your partner.

- Breakage, though infrequent, can happen; most studies reveal that breakage occurs in only one or two condoms out of one hundred.
- Some men cannot maintain an erection with condoms or experience a reduction in sensation; textured, ultrathin, or transparent condoms can help.

Tips for Smart Sex

To be most effective, condoms should be used with a spermicidal foam, cream, or jelly. These products can be inserted into the vagina before intercourse. Or a small amount of spermicide can be placed inside the condom before it is rolled on as well as on the outside surface of the condom after it is in place. If a condom breaks during sex, immediately insert additional spermicide into the vagina. Never reuse condoms, and avoid contact with oil-based products—such as Vaseline, hand lotion, or even yeast infection creams—which can erode the latex. Keep condoms in a cool, dark place, and never use a condom after its expiration date.

About condoms and talcum powder: Putting talc into your underwear has been shown to increase your risk of developing ovarian cancer. No one knows whether the talc that's on condoms also poses a threat to your reproductive health. Even so, some doctors have asked condom manufacturers to reduce or eliminate talc from their products. In the meantime, it may make sense to use talc-free or low-talc brands.

The Feel-Good Factor

Often incorporated into sex play, condoms may enhance a man's erection—the rim of the condom traps the blood in the penis, keeping it engorged and rigid. New research shows that use of a water-based lubricant decreases the chance of condom breakage (it may also increase stimulation for both partners).

The Female Condom

The Basics

The polyurethane female condom, brand name Reality, is inserted into a woman's vagina before genital contact. Reality has two rings that help hold the condom in place. The inner ring, which is similar to the rim of the diaphragm, is squeezed together and pushed into the vagina, then placed near the cervical opening. The outer ring stays outside the vagina, partially covering the vulva (external genitals).

Failure rate: 5 percent perfect use, 21 percent typical use.

Cost: about $10 for a package of three.

Ideal User

Reality is best for women who wish to have control over contraception and protect themselves from disease as well as pregnancy. Like users of the male condom, Reality users don't have to worry about long-term health consequences.

Pros

- The female condom may be more protective against some STDs than the male condom because it keeps the skin around the opening of the vagina from coming into contact with the penis.
- Users do not have to wait for a partner's erection to put it on, thus it is less likely to interrupt foreplay than the male condom.
- Reality is made of durable polyurethane, so people who are allergic to latex can use it safely—and polyurethane has a longer shelf life than latex condoms.
- In a recent study comparing male and female condoms, users preferred Reality.
- Has been approved for Medicaid reimbursement in nearly forty states.
- Can be put into place up to eight hours prior to intercourse.

Cons

- Reality is not as effective as the male condom, and its effectiveness is somewhat lower than several other methods of contraception in preventing pregnancy.
- Some users say Reality is baggy and squeaky.
- Reality has a public relations problem: People aren't trying it because it's unfamiliar.

Tips for Smart Sex

Although the female condom was designed and tested for use without spermicide, Reality can be used with a spermicide to improve its effectiveness. You can place spermicide in the vagina prior to insertion of the condom or insert it directly into the condom. Any lubricant can be used with the female condom because oil-based products will not erode polyurethane. As with traditional condoms, you should never reuse the female condom, and do not use it past the expiration date on the packaging. Store it at room temperature.

The Feel-Good Factor

The outer ring of the device, which helps keep it in place, is thought to increase clitoral stimulation in some users.

The Pill

The Basics

Most oral contraceptives contain estrogen and progestin, a synthetic version of the naturally occurring hormone progesterone. The estrogen works by suppressing ovulation or preventing the ovaries from releasing an egg. The progestin helps to thicken the cervical mucus, foiling the movement of sperm. Pills that contain both estrogen and progestin are also referred to as combined oral contraceptives.

Failure rate: 0.1 percent perfect use, 5 percent typical use.

Cost: $100 to $300 per year.

Ideal User

Savvy, sexually active women who can remember to take a pill every day—preferably at the same time of day (try associating it with a routine task, like brushing your teeth).

Pros

- Extremely effective at preventing pregnancy.
- Reversible; no loss of fertility.
- Doesn't interfere with foreplay or lovemaking.
- It's safe—can be used cumulatively and consistently throughout the reproductive years.
- Makes periods more regular, less painful, and lighter.
- Protects against certain cancers, pelvic inflammatory disease (PID), noncancerous breast tumors, and ovarian cysts. Also protects against ectopic (tubal) pregnancies. *(See "Reconsidering the Pill," page 56.)*
- May be used to treat or prevent endometriosis.

Cons

- Pills must be taken every day.
- Somewhat expensive; insurance is unlikely to cover the cost, unless prescribed for use other than contraception.
- Possible side effects include irregular, scanty bleeding and spotting.
- Less common side effects include headaches, nausea during the first pill cycle, depression, pregnancy "mask" (places of darkened pigment on the face, especially the forehead), and an increased risk for urinary tract infections.
- Smokers over the age of thirty-five on the Pill appear to have a greater risk for heart disease, blood clots, or stroke.

- Occasional missed periods disturb some women.
- Provides no STD protection.

Tips for Smart Sex

For best results, use a backup method of birth control *for seven days* when you have missed a pill (especially near the beginning of the cycle) and *for the rest of the month* if you have an episode of vomiting or diarrhea because under these conditions the Pill may not have the opportunity to get into your system. Antiseizure medications, barbiturates (Phenobarbital), and some antibiotics (penicillin, tetracycline) may sabotage the Pill, so whenever you are prescribed a new drug, remind the doctor that you're on oral contraceptives.

The Feel-Good Factor

Pill users often report increased sexual pleasure, probably due to freedom from pregnancy worries. In a recent study from San Francisco State University, users of so-called triphasic oral contraceptives—in which the progestin dose varies throughout the month—reported having more vaginal lubrication and greater sexual interest and satisfaction than users of monophasic pills (in which the progestin dose is constant).

Some women experience lowered libido after going on oral contraceptives. Alert your physician if you notice a change in your sex drive. It may be possible to switch to a different formulation that does not interfere with sexual desire.

The Mini-Pill

The Basics

The mini-pill contains progestin, which primarily works by thickening the cervical mucus, slowing sperm to a crawl.

Failure rate: .5 percent perfect use, 6 percent typical use.

Cost: $100 to $300 per year.

Ideal User

Women who like the freedom of oral contraceptives and have the discipline to take a pill each day *at the same time of day.* The mini-pill is particularly unforgiving when not taken as directed. Women in the latter part of their reproductive years are prime candidates because the mini-pill is more effective in older women.

55

Pros

- Reversible. No loss of fertility.
- Doesn't interfere with foreplay or lovemaking.
- Like combined pills, it can be safely used throughout the reproductive years.
- Makes periods more regular, less painful, and lighter.
- May be useful against endometriosis.
- Provides similar health benefits as the combined pill.
- Mini-pill provides a hormonal alternative to women who cannot take estrogen.
- Mini-pill can also be used by lactating women. (Combined pills can diminish the quantity of milk produced.)

Cons

- Mini-pill users must be diligent.
- Somewhat expensive.
- Likely to produce irregular, scanty bleeding and spotting.
- Both weight gain and breast tenderness are common.
- Mini-pill increases the risk for ovarian cysts.
- Provides no STD protection.

Tips for Smart Sex

The mini-pill should be taken at the same time of day and a backup method used for two days if you are more than two hours late, according to James Trussell, Ph.D., director of population research at Princeton University. If you have an episode of vomiting or diarrhea, use the backup method along with the mini-pill until two days after you are well again. Antiseizure medications, barbiturates (Phenobarbital), and some antibiotics (penicillin, tetracycline) may sabotage the mini-pill, so when you are prescribed a new drug, remind your doctor that you're on oral contraceptives.

The Feel-Good Factor

Some women experience lowered libido after going on the mini-pill. Alert your physician if you notice a change in your sex drive.

Reconsidering the Pill

More than 17 million American women use birth control pills—and oral contraceptives are second only to sterilization in popularity among contraceptive users. With those kinds of numbers, it's hard to imagine that the Pill ever had a public relations problem.

When it was introduced in 1960, the Pill promised women virtual freedom from pregnancy worries for the first time in history. By the 1970s and 80s, however, other big worries had surfaced: links to heart disease, stroke, and breast cancer.

Today oral contraceptives have been nearly redeemed. The Pill is one of the most studied medications around, and volumes of data link it to numerous health *benefits,* including protection against some deadly cancers, and establish its safety for women throughout their reproductive years. It appears that many of the health problems associated with Pill use often relate to high-risk behaviors like smoking.

But the biggest concern for potential Pill users is the reputed link to breast cancer. Until recently the data associating pill use and breast cancer risk were not completely clear-cut. "There was no fire, but a lot of smoke," says Carolyn Westhoff, M.D., associate professor of obstetrics and gynecology at Columbia Presbyterian Medical Center. "The studies tended to be weak or inconclusive."

Small wonder that many women remain confused—and suspicious. Knowing the facts about the Pill should help you make an informed decision about whether or not it's right for you.

Not Your Mother's Birth Control Pill

The first thing you should know is that the Pill has changed, according to Susan Wysocki, R.N.C., N.P., president of the National Association of Nurse-Practitioners in Reproductive Health. When oral contraceptives were first introduced, most versions contained 10 milligrams of progestin (the synthetic version of the naturally occurring hormone, progesterone) and 150 milligrams of estrogen. Most of today's pills have one tenth the amount of progestin (1 milligram) and one fourth the estrogen (35 milligrams). "We didn't realize we were overdosing women," says Elizabeth B. Connell, M.D., professor in the Department of Gynecology and Obstetrics at Emory University School of Medicine in Atlanta and an early Pill researcher. Many of the health problems associated with the early Pill were related to these high hormone levels.

Cardiovascular Disease: The early Pill increased a woman's chance of developing blood clots, heart attack, or stroke. Today's lower dose pills do not increase a woman's risk of heart attack and stroke *unless she smokes.* (A fifteen-cigarette-a-day habit results in a twenty-one-fold increase in these cardiovascular risks.)

Breast Cancer: Increasingly the data suggest that birth control pills do not pose a breast cancer risk. The latest evidence: a huge multistudy analysis conducted by researchers from twenty-five countries that examined fifty-four epidemiological studies involving more than 60,000 women. The new study—conducted by researchers at Oxford University—found that ten years after going off birth control pills, women who had used them were at no greater risk for breast cancer than women who had not used them. It didn't matter what a woman's age was when she started and stopped the Pill, the number of years on it, whether she had a family history of breast cancer, or the type and dose of pill used. "This should lay the matter to rest," Westhoff says.

According to the study, current Pill users may have a higher rate of breast cancer *diagnosis,* but it is probably related to regularity of health care. "When women are getting regular checkups, there are more opportunities for diagnosis," Westhoff says. "Women on the Pill have regular contact with health-care facilities."

"Third-Generation" Pills and Blood Clots: Recent studies conducted in England shed a negative light on so-called "third-generation" oral contraceptives. These pills contain new kinds of progestin (artificial progesterone). These types of progestin are rare in this country (Ortho-Cept or Desogen are the only third-generation brands sold in the United States) but are favored by many European women because they are less likely to trigger unpleasant side effects such as acne or an increase in the growth of facial hair. The new data suggest that the third-generation pills increase the risk of developing potentially fatal blood clots. The increase is real, though small, so if you are on either brand, ask your doctor to help you assess the possible risks. Women who are overweight are not advised to take them.

Reproductive Tract Cancers: Studies indicate that the Pill protects against endometrial and ovarian cancers. A woman taking the Pill has a 40 to 60 percent lower risk of developing ovarian cancer, a rare but deadly disease. And the protection increases over time. Pill users decrease their risk of endometrial cancer by half. Protection against both cancers lasts at least fifteen years after a woman stops taking the Pill.

The Pill's relationship to cervical cancer is unclear, although some studies show that oral contraceptives enhance the risk for the disease. But this link may be influenced by other factors. Pill users tend to have sex more frequently, for instance, increasing the chance of contracting human papilloma virus, which is linked to cervical cancer. Women on birth control pills are also more likely to get regular Pap smears, which may increase the detection of cervical cancer.

Other Health Benefits: Pill use diminishes the incidence of benign breast lumps and ovarian cysts and decreases the risk for pelvic inflammatory disease (PID), perhaps by thickening the cervical mucus, which hampers the movement of microbes in the reproductive tract. In this fashion it may help protect fertility, since PID can impair a woman's ability to conceive a child. Oral contraceptives also reduce the incidence of ectopic pregnancies. And they may help shore up bone mass during perimenopause (the period just prior to menopause) when bone loss tends to accelerate.

Who Can Take the Pill

Most healthy women can take the Pill safely. The American College of Obstetricians and Gynecologists has now declared oral contraceptives to be safe for women over the age of thirty-five. And in 1990 the FDA cleared the way for drug companies to state on their labeling that the pill's benefits may outweigh the possible risks for healthy nonsmoking women over age forty. In fact, an increasing number of practitioners are prescribing oral contraceptives to help ease women through the transition to menopause, which is often marked by hot flashes and irregular bleeding, says Valerie Montgomery Rice, M.D., a reproductive endocrinologist at the University of Kansas Medical Center in Lawrence. Taking the Pill helps reduce the severity of these problems.

Some health-care providers believe that the Pill is safe for younger women (under age thirty-five) who smoke, though they may skirt the issue because they don't wish to be seen as endorsing this negative behavior. If you smoke, tell your doctor—being honest about smoking or other health-related behaviors is the only way your physician can properly advise you about any drug or medical treatment.

Who Should Not Take the Pill

You should not take oral contraceptives if you:

- have a history of heart disease, stroke, or any blood-clotting disorder
- have had breast or endometrial cancer or liver disease
- smoke and are over the age of thirty-five.

The Diaphragm

The Basics

The diaphragm is a shallow, dome-shaped rubber cup with a flexible rim that fits in the vagina, blocking the cervix. Spermicide is placed inside the diaphragm prior to insertion and reapplied with each act of intercourse. The device can be inserted up to six hours before sex and must be left in place for at least six hours after intercourse.

Failure rate: 6 percent perfect use, 18 percent typical use.

Cost: About $20 plus the cost of the initial examination and spermicide (about 25¢ per use).

Ideal User

The diaphragm is best for women in stable, monogamous relationships who want a good reversible method of birth control and who can't or don't want to use hormone-based methods.

Pros

- Provides protection against some STDs, including gonorrhea and chlamydia and PID (which can lead to infertility), although it does not protect against AIDS.
- May reduce the risk of developing cervical cancer.
- If inserted in advance, need not interfere with foreplay.

Cons

- Inconvenient and difficult for some women to insert.
- Must be refitted every two years.
- May become dislodged when the woman is on top during intercourse.
- Bladder infections are a problem for some users.
- In rare cases, the diaphragm has been associated with toxic shock syndrome. (Symptoms include sudden high fever, diarrhea, vomiting, sore throat, aching muscles and joints, dizziness or faintness, and rash. *For more information about toxic shock syndrome, see page 47.*)
- Some women are allergic to rubber.

Tips for Smart Sex

As long as you use your diaphragm diligently and correctly, it's unlikely to disappoint you. For best results, have the device fitted around the time of ovulation to insure a proper fit; the cervix changes shape during the cycle and is most dilated at ovulation. You need to be refitted if you lose or gain more than ten pounds and after childbirth.

Check the device for holes *every few weeks*. Avoid touching the device with talcum powder or oil-based products (Vaseline, hand lotion, soaps like Dove, many yeast infection creams), which can erode the rubber. Wash your hands before you insert the diaphragm. If the device becomes dislodged during sex, insert additional spermicide with the applicator, removing the plunger carefully so the spermicide doesn't retract back into the applicator.

The Feel-Good Factor

The diaphragm can be inserted well before sex, so it need not spoil your intimate moments. During oral sex, some men may be aware of and not like the taste of spermicides.

The Cervical Cap

The Basics

Similar to the diaphragm but smaller. Fits snugly over the cervix and must be left in place for at least eight hours after intercourse. It can be left in place up to forty-eight hours. The cap should be filled up one-third with spermicide before inserting.

Failure rate (in women who have not had children): 9 percent perfect use, 18 percent typical use. (The failure rate is higher in women who have had children, perhaps because it is more likely to become dislodged from the cervix after childbirth.)

Cost: Same as diaphragm.

Ideal User

Users like its relative lack of health risks or side effects. Because you can insert it and leave it in for up to forty-eight hours, the cap provides some measure of sexual spontaneity. However, it only comes in four sizes (not everyone will be a fit), and it seems to work best in women who have never had a baby. You must keep it scrupulously clean to prevent bacterial buildup and odor.

Pros

- May protect against some STDs, including gonorrhea, chlamydia, and PID (not AIDS).
- Reduces risk of cervical cancer.

- Since it can be inserted eight hours prior to intercourse, it is unlikely to interfere with lovemaking.

Cons

- Abnormal cell growth occur in the cervix during the first few months of use, possibly due to the cap making the cervix more vulnerable to human papilloma virus (*see chapter 2, page 14*). (Women must get a Pap smear before using the cap and again three months later. If the follow-up test shows abnormal cells, cap use must be discontinued.)
- May cause irritation.
- May slightly increase the risk of toxic shock syndrome. (*For more information, see pp. 47.*)
- Some women are allergic to rubber.
- Cap can develop an odor.

Tips for Smart Sex

For best results, check the cap for holes *every* time you use it. As with the diaphragm, talcum powder and oil-based products can erode the rubber.

Have the cap fitted around the time of ovulation, when the cervix is most dilated. Although the cap's instructions suggest that one dose of spermicide is all that's needed while you are wearing it, inserting more with each act of intercourse will increase your margin of safety, advises Samuel A. Pasquale, M.D., chief of women's health research at Robert Woods Johnson Medical School in New Jersey. Remember to remove the plunger without tugging on it, which can remove the spermicide. If the cap becomes dislodged during sex, insert additional spermicide.

The Feel-Good Factor

Since it can be put in place hours before intercourse, the cap is less likely to put a damper on foreplay and lovemaking. During oral sex, men are unlikely to be aware of spermicides because the cap fits snugly over the cervix, keeping spermicides trapped inside.

Norplant

The Basics

Norplant consists of six silicone capsules placed under the skin in the upper arm. The capsules, or rods, slow-release synthetic progesterone for five years.

Failure rate: .09 percent perfect use, .09 percent typical use.

Cost: $500 to $700.

Ideal User

If you're at the peak of fertility and a low-maintenance type, this five-year contraceptive plan could be right for you. The downside is the possibility of irregular bleeding and headaches. Some users have had trouble with removal, but clinicians have been improving the procedure so as to reduce pain and scarring.

Norplant is also good if you have a medical condition that could harm a fetus or you have completed childbearing but are not ready for or don't want permanent sterilization.

Pros

- Prevents pregnancy for five years.
- Complete contraception freedom: nothing to remember, nothing to insert.
- Can be used by women who cannot tolerate estrogen-based oral contraceptives.
- Long-term but reversible.

Cons

- Side effects include irregular bleeding to no periods, headaches, depression, and weight gain.
- A medical procedure is needed to insert and remove Norplant.
- Women sometimes get an infection at the site of insertion.
- Not effective against STDs.
- May reduce sex drive.

Tips for Smart Sex

Use a backup birth control method during the first twenty-four hours of use, and have the rods replaced on schedule. Remember to use a condom for STD protection. Antiseizure drugs and rifampin, an antituberculosis drug, can reduce Norplant's effectiveness. The skill and experience of the practitioner is important in using this method; don't hesitate to ask your health-care provider about his experience with inserting and removing the rods.

The Feel-Good Factor

Nearly complete freedom from pregnancy concerns is likely to boost your sexual pleasure, unless the progesterone lulls your libido, a possible adverse side effect.

Depo-Provera

The Basics

Depo Provera is an injection of progesterone that works by suppressing ovulation, thickening cervical mucus, and preventing a fertilized egg from implanting in the uterus. One injection is good for three months.

Failure rate: .3 percent perfect use, .3 typical use.

Cost: $30 to $75 per injection.

Ideal User

Women who cannot remember to take a daily pill but who want a hormonal contraception. Depo Provera offers considerable contraceptive freedom for the small price of getting quarterly injections.

Pros

- Prevents pregnancy for twelve weeks.
- No daily pills, nothing to insert.
- Can be used by women who are breastfeeding (mothers must wait six weeks after delivery).
- Some women who cannot take the Pill can tolerate Depo Provera.
- Protects against cancer of the lining of the uterus and anemia (iron deficiency).

Cons

- Side effects include irregular periods or none at all. Less common: headaches, hair loss, weight gain, depression, and abdominal pain.
- Side effects continue for the duration of the method's effective period.
- Return to fertility may be delayed. (The median time for conceiving after discontinuing Depo Provera is six months.)
- Not effective against STDs.
- May reduce sex drive.

Tips for Smart Sex

For best results, use an additional contraceptive for the first two weeks after the injection. Use a backup contraception if your doctor prescribes drugs that can diminish Depo Provera's effectiveness (antiseizure drugs or rifampin, an antituberculosis drug). Return for injections on schedule. Use a condom to protect yourself against STDs.

The Feel-Good Factor

Like Norplant, Depo Provera's high effectiveness often gives users contraceptive confidence, which may translate into a greater ability to surrender to erotic pleasure. Some users may experience a reduction in sexual desire, though.

The IUD

The Basics

The IUD is a small T-shaped device that's placed in the uterus. It prevents fertilization by inactivating either the egg or the sperm (how is not exactly known). Researchers used to believe that IUDs hindered the implantation of a fertilized egg. Current research suggests that they may work by immobilizing sperm or speeding the egg through the fallopian tube before it can become fertilized. There are two types available in the United States—the ParaGard T (Ortho Pharmaceuticals), which is made of plastic and has copper as its active ingredient, and Progestasert (Alza Corp.), which contains progesterone. Both types have monofilament threads, or strings, that you can check periodically to make sure the IUD is in place.

Failure rate: .1 to 1.5 perfect use, 0.1 to 2 percent typical use.

Cost: $200 to $300 (including exam cost).

Ideal User

Monogamy and motherhood make good IUD matches. Having more than one sex partner puts you at greater risk for STDs, a special concern for IUD users. If you've ever given birth, your uterus will be more receptive to the device, and you will be less likely to expel it.

Women who use IUDs have an increased risk for pelvic inflammatory disease (PID), so if you have ever had an STD, you are not a good candidate for the device. Because of the enhanced risk of pelvic infections—and the infertility that can then result—the IUD is most often prescribed to women who have completed their childbearing. It is usually not prescribed to women with fibroids or women who have had an ectopic pregnancy. An IUD is also a good method for women whose periods are light and fairly painless, which decreases the chance of expulsion.

Pros

- Less expensive than any other form of birth control, since it is good for a number of years.
- Women who can't or don't want to use hormonal methods can use it successfully.
- Complete contraceptive freedom for up to ten years.
- It is reversible.

Cons

- Carries higher risk for PID and other infections, particularly in the time period immediately following insertion. (Antibiotics are often prescribed to prevent infection at the time of insertion.)
- Users often report greater menstrual bleeding and cramping. (The progesterone-releasing IUD may decrease bleeding and cramps.)
- There is a 2 to 10 percent chance of expulsion in the first year, especially among younger users and those with a history of heavy menstrual blood flow and cramping.
- Half of pregnancies that do occur with the IUD in place end in spontaneous abortion; a small percentage of pregnancies that occur with the device are ectopic pregnancies.
- Must be inserted and removed by a physician.

Tips for Smart Sex

One of the most carefree methods around for those who can use it, the IUD is good for years. Simply check the strings frequently during the first month of use and regularly after each menstrual period. Replace on schedule if the IUD contains progesterone.

The Feel-Good Factor

The IUD will keep you worry free, enhancing your time spent between the sheets. It is unlikely to interfere with your libido.

The Dalkon Shield Debacle

In the 1970s, a fish-shaped IUD called the Dalkon Shield was introduced to the market. It contributed to thousands of miscarriages and even some deaths among American women. Lawsuits drove the company out of business and convinced many women and physicians that IUDs were unsafe. Many doctors still do not prescribe IUDs. Contraceptive experts generally agree, however, that the types that are currently available are safe and effective. "It's the single most effective reversible method of birth control—and highly underused," says James Trussell, Ph.D., director of population research at Princeton University.

Sterilization

The Basics

One of the safest and most cost effective methods of birth control, sterilization involves blocking the fallopian tubes to prevent sperm and egg from uniting. (The male version—the vasectomy—blocks the vas deferens to prevent the sperm from passing into the ejaculate.)

Failure rate:

Female sterilization: .4 perfect use, .4 typical use

Male sterilization: .10 perfect use, .15 typical use

Cost: $1,500 to $2,500 (female); $250 to $1,000 (male)

Ideal User

Women who have ended their childbearing or who know with certainty that they do not want children.

Pros

- Permanent, safe, and highly effective.
- No long-term side effects.
- No pills to take, nothing to insert or remember.
- Partner's cooperation is not required.

Cons

- Requires surgical procedure and, thus, has a certain amount of risk.
- No protection against STDs.
- Not easily reversed.

Tips for Smart Sex

Sterilization is not completely foolproof. Pregnancies are extremely rare, but when they do occur, they often result in ectopic pregnancies, so it's wise to be alert to the possible signs. Alert your doctor if you have sudden intense pain in the lower abdomen, irregular bleeding or spotting with abdominal pain when your period is late, fainting, or dizziness that persists for more than a few seconds. Use a condom to protect yourself against STDs.

If your partner has had a vasectomy, it's important to remember that he is not sterile immediately. Sperm is not cleared from the reproductive tract until approximately fifteen ejaculations, according to *Contraceptive Technology*. In the meantime, use a backup method of birth control, and have the doctor examine your partner's semen after fifteen ejaculations to be sure you are safe.

The Feel-Good Factor

Sterilization offers the most effective form of contraception, so concerns about pregnancy are a thing of the past.

Developed in China, the new "no-scalpel" vasectomy has been in use in the United States for several years. It offers some attractive advantages over the traditional procedure. In a conventional vasectomy, the doctor makes one or two small incisions in the skin and cuts the vas deferens, the tubes that transport sperm from the testicles to the penis. Using the no-scalpel technique, the doctor makes a tiny puncture with a special instrument, then blocks the vas deferens using the same technique as conventional vasectomy. No stitches are necessary to close the puncture. The simpler technique is associated with reduced pain and bleeding, a shorter recovery time, and fewer complications than the traditional vasectomy.

Considering Vasectomy

If you and your partner are certain you do not want more children—or any at all—sterilization is a good option. Both vasectomy and tubal sterilization are nearly 100 percent effective in preventing pregnancy, but if you look at the choice in terms of cost, convenience, and safety, vasectomy is the preferred method of sterilization. Only you and your partner can make the decision. Here's a comparison of the two methods:

VASECTOMY VS. TUBAL STERILIZATION		
Procedure	Vasectomy	Tubal Ligation
Surgery	Performed in a doctor's office under local anesthesia	Done in an operating room under general anesthesia
Complications	Mild discomfort and swelling	Possible pain at the site of the incision; soreness from carbon dioxide pumped into abdomen
Cost	$250 to $1,000	$1,500 to $2,500
Recovery	48 hours	2 weeks

Contraception to Go: Spermicidal Foams, Creams, Jellies, Suppositories, and Film

The Basics

Over-the-counter vaginal spermicides are among the easiest contraceptives to obtain. Most of these products contain the chemicals nonoxynol-9 or octoxynol, which kill sperm. They are either used alone or with a barrier contraceptive such as a diaphragm or condom. One of the newest products, contraceptive film—translucent 2.4-inch squares (they resemble soap leaves)—can be conveniently stashed in a back pocket or purse.

Failure rate: 6 percent perfect use, 21 percent typical use.

Cost: 35¢ to $12.

Ideal User

Products like foam and suppositories are often favored by people who don't use contraception on a regular basis, who need a stopgap between methods, or who want an adjunct or backup to other methods.

Pros

- No doctor visit is necessary.
- Women can use them without their partner's involvement or knowledge.
- They can be a backup if a condom breaks during intercourse.

Cons

- Although in test-tube studies spermicides appear to kill many of the organisms that cause STDs—including AIDS—their record with people who are actually having sex is mixed. *They have not been endorsed as effective protection against STDs.* Some research demonstrated that spermicidal suppositories decreased the transmission of HIV, but one study showed the sponges containing a spermicide actually increased the chances for infection.
- Spermicides are irritating to some women and may disrupt the normal flora in the vagina, triggering infections.

Tips for Smart Sex

To increase the effectiveness of spermicides against disease and pregnancy, use them with a condom. Get familiar with the instructions on the product packaging well before sex and follow them carefully. Use the recommended amount of spermicide with each act of intercourse. Suppositories and film must have adequate time to dissolve, usually ten minutes. Shake foaming agents well before inserting. Spermicides often lose their effectiveness after an hour, so be prepared to apply more, even if you have not yet had intercourse.

The Feel-Good Factor

Over-the-counter methods are good for sexual spontaneity. If you choose and use them wisely, spermicides can keep you safe and sexy.

Rhythm Revised

What if someone offered you a method of birth control that was effective and inexpensive, required no device, did not interfere with the act of intercourse or disrupt your body's natural hormone balance, had no side effects, increased your body awareness, and enhanced communication between you and your partner? You'd probably say, "Great—sign me up."

Now, what if you learned that the method involved daily monitoring and required periods of abstinence (no intercourse) or use of another method during your monthly fertile periods? You'd then likely say, "Not so fast."

Natural birth control—popularly called "fertility awareness" (there are several related methods)—involves identifying the times of the cycle when your body is fertile and avoiding intercourse during them. It should not be confused with the rhythm method, which is notoriously ineffective.

For the record, the rhythm, or calendar, method—which was developed around 1930—involves tracking the length of a woman's menstrual cycle for a year, then applying simple mathematics to arrive at a first and last "safe" day for sexual intercourse. It deals with averages and is therefore unreliable because a woman's cycle can vary from month to month. In fact, the rhythm method has a whopping failure rate of 30 percent.

The newer methods of natural birth control take advantage of medicine's increased understanding of reproductive physiology. Just prior to ovulation, estrogen causes the cervical mucus to become more elastic, which makes it easier for sperm to penetrate the cervix. The consistency of the mucus is often compared to raw egg whites. (The mucus also forms a fernlike pattern when dried and viewed on a microscope slide.) After ovulation, progesterone kicks in, altering the mucus yet again and reducing sperm movement to a crawl. The surge in progesterone also triggers a slight increase in body temperature.

Fertility awareness requires time and discipline. But if practiced diligently, it offers an effectiveness rate comparable to the male condom and the diaphragm. In a recent analysis of several studies conducted around the world during the 1990s, researchers found that pregnancy rates varied from 1.7 to 10.6 (per one hundred women during the first year), placing it on a par with many forms of birth control popular with American women.

Fertility awareness methods have been used by women from India to Belgium, Germany, Liberia, Zambia, the United Kingdom, and many other parts of the globe. Researchers who have studied it frequently chalk up its failures to imperfect use.

Fertility awareness and the body wisdom it confers provide some nifty perks besides pregnancy prevention. If you commit to it, you join a community of women worldwide who are uniquely in touch with their bodies and their cycles. Practicing these methods can also alert you to subtle health clues that may signal illness. "One of the benefits is that women learn what is a completely normal cycle for them, so they know if there's something out of line," says Toni Weschler, M.P.H., a health educator and author of *Taking Charge of Your Fertility.*

Fertility awareness also fosters intimacy and communication between you and your partner. Many partners participate in the process by helping women maintain their charts or taking their temperature in the morning. And when you're ready for pregnancy, fertility awareness can help you pinpoint the best time to conceive (*see "Conscious Conception," page 78*).

The Basics

There are two natural birth control methods in wide use. The Billings Ovulation Method, developed by Australian physicians John and Lyn Billings, relies only on the consistency and other characteristics of the cervical mucus. Couples use a chart to monitor mucus changes during the entire cycle. The peak mucus sign is considered to be the last day that cervical mucus is clear and stretchy (you can often stretch it several inches between your index finger and thumb). The infertile period begins on the fourth day after this mucus peak. Using the Symptothermal Method, women take their temperature using an ovulation or "basal" thermometer each morning before they get up. In most women, body temperature falls slightly just before ovulation and rises again just after ovulation, so you can learn to estimate the time of ovulation. You also assess the cervical mucus and watch for other signs of ovulation: breast tenderness, abdominal pain, back pain, and mood changes, for example.

Failure rate: 2 to 3 percent perfect use; typical use unknown.

Cots: Fees for counseling services and start-up costs (charts, thermometers) vary significantly; backup methods used during fertile times also varies.

Ideal User

Fertility awareness is for women who have the willingness and patience to become familiar with their body's natural cycles and who appreciate the sexual freedom possible during their nonfertile times.

Pros

- Requires no chemicals.
- No side effects.
- Appropriate for women who cannot use hormonal methods of birth control.
- Highly effective if used correctly and consistently.
- Provides body knowledge that can help you stay healthy.

- Significant emotional and psychological benefits.
- Enhanced communication with partner.

Cons

- Requires dedication and diligence.
- Periods of abstinence a drawback for some women.
- Some women have a continuous or variable presence of mucus or bleed irregularly, which can make testing the mucus more difficult. Semen in the vagina can also obscure the mucus test.
- Some women do not show the classic dip and rise in body temperature at ovulation. Illness (especially when accompanied by fever), use of drugs—such as aspirin and alcohol—sleeplessness, stress, and travel can affect the accuracy of your chart keeping.
- Fertility awareness is complicated. To be effective, these methods require following detailed instruction best learned from an expert in this method of natural birth control.

Tips for Safe Sex

It is strongly advised that you seek assistance from an organization that offers training in fertility awareness methods (*see "Resources," page 87*). Many of these organizations will put you in touch with an instructor in your area.

Use a backup method of birth control on the days that you have determined you are fertile. For best results, continue to chart your symptoms and temperature each day even if you think you know when you are ovulating.

The Feel-Good Factor

With fertility awareness, nothing comes between you and your partner. What could be better for your sex life?

Men and Contraception

Contraception has a history of being the woman's worry. For good reason: Females pay a greater price for unplanned pregnancies. But a 1997 survey conducted by the Kaiser Family Foundation suggests that women may be selling their men short. For instance, the data show that a majority of men think they should be playing a greater role in contraceptive decisions, and close to a third report feeling left out of the process. Eighty percent of the men questioned acknowledge that women feel more responsibility about birth control. But many of them say they want to be more involved; some say they would be willing to use a male method if better ones were available. Two-thirds of men, for example, say they would themselves consider taking a hormonal contraceptive. "This indicates an opportunity for men to play a more significant role in reproductive decision-making, a role many seem willing to take on," says Felicia H. Stewart, M.D., director of reproductive health programs for the Kaiser Family Foundation.

Even if men don't use the methods themselves, there are other ways for them to take responsibility for contraceptive decisions. They can, for instance, insist that contraception be used during each act of intercourse or help their partners to remember to use birth control correctly.

Before they can be a part of contraceptive decisions and practices, however, men will first have to catch up on the current options: More than half admit they do not know much about the available methods, and a full one in five knows next to nothing about birth control.

Birth Control: What's Hot, What's Not

About 38 million American women use some form of birth control or have been sterilized (or have partners who have been sterilized), according to the Alan Guttmacher Institute. Some contraceptive methods are more popular than others. Here's how the numbers break down:

Method	Percentage of Users
Tubal Ligation	27.7
Pill	26.9
Male Condom	20.4
Vasectomy	10.9
Withdrawal	3.0
Depo Provera	3.0
Periodic Abstinence	2.3
Diaphragm	1.9
Other Methods	1.8
Norplant	1.3
IUD	0.8
Total percentage	100

Source: "Fertility, Family Planning, and Women's Health: New Data from the 1995 National Survey of Family Growth," Vital and Health Statistics, Series 23, No. 19, May 1997, CDC, NCHS.

Morning-After Birth Control

It's a nightmare. You are the victim of a sexual assault.

Or your best intentions go awry when the condom breaks during sex.

While these scenarios are not pleasant to think about, devoting attention to them now could save you considerable worry in the future. Whether your birth control fails or you fail to use birth control, there is a solution: emergency contraception.

Emergency contraception refers to methods of birth control that are either taken (oral contraceptives, mini-pills) or inserted (the copper IUD) after unprotected intercourse to prevent conception. Morning-after methods of birth control are cheap and effective and have minimal side effects. They should not be confused with abortion: Both pills and the IUD alter the uterine lining and interfere with implantation and fertilization; they do not abort a fetus.

When should you consider emergency birth control? According to *Contraceptive Technology,* an authoritative sexual health book for health professionals:

- You were forced to have sex.
- A condom broke or slipped off.
- You didn't use any birth control.
- Your diaphragm slipped out of place.
- You had sex when you didn't expect it.
- You stopped taking birth control pills for more than a week.
- You missed as many as half of your birth control pills in the past two weeks.

Although health-care practitioners have known about "after-the-fact" contraception for two decades—some university health-care facilities have offered it quietly to students for years—data show that many women still do not know about it, and doctors rarely inform their patients about this option. A survey conducted by the Kaiser Family Foundation found that only one-third of American women know that anything can be done after unprotected sex to prevent pregnancy. The same survey revealed that doctors use these methods five or fewer times a year and often make patients aware of them only in response to emergency situations rather than during contraceptive counseling.

In other words, you have to know about it to ask for it.

The price for this communication gap is staggering: The authors of *Contraceptive Technology* estimate that emergency contraception could reduce by 1.7 million the number of unintended pregnancies each year, and reduce the number of abortions by 800,000.

One reason more women don't know about postcoital contraception is that these contraceptive methods have not been approved for this use. To gain approval, manufacturers of birth control pills and IUDs would have to petition the FDA to add emergency contraception to package labeling.

It is legal for doctors to prescribe drugs and medical products already on the market for uses other than what they were approved. For example, oral contraceptives are routinely prescribed for such "off-label" uses as regulating menstrual periods, preventing the recurrence of ovarian cysts, treating endometriosis, and reducing acne. In 1998, Gynetics Inc. of Somerville, New Jersey, plans to market emergency contraception pills packaged for this purpose.

How It Works

Emergency contraceptive pills are ordinary oral contraceptives (which combine estrogen and synthetic progesterone) that can be taken up to seventy-two hours after the unprotected sexual episode. The second option is the progesterone-only "mini-pill," which can be taken up to forty-eight hours afterward. Both are followed by a second dose twelve hours later. The pill methods are 75 percent effective in preventing pregnancy. Nausea and/or vomiting is common when using the combined pills, so some doctors also prescribe Dramamine to reduce this side effect.

The third option is a copper IUD, which can be inserted *up to seven days* after unprotected sex. It is advised only for women who will continue to use the IUD, so generally you must be a good candidate for the method. (*See "The IUD," page 65.*)

The hormone regimens that can be used for emergency contraception

PILL	ONE DOSE EQUALS:
Ovral	Two white pills
Levlen	Four light-orange pills
Lo/Ovral	Four white pills
Nordette	Four light-orange pills
Triphasil	Four yellow pills
Tri-Levlen	Four yellow pills
Alesse	Five pink pills
Ovrette (mini-pill)	Twenty yellow pills

are found in certain brand-name pills (see previous page). If you are already on one of these pills, keep an extra pack around for the unexpected. Generally, however, it is best to discuss the methods and doses with your doctor because pill regimens can change. Ask your health-care provider about emergency contraception during your annual exam; he may prescribe pills to keep on hand for emergencies—even if you are not a regular pill user.

If you use pills, take them with food to minimize the chance of nausea, and call your doctor if you throw up because an additional dose may be necessary. Also alert your doctor if you develop any of the following symptoms, which may signal the very rare possibility that the treatment triggered a stroke:

- severe leg pain
- severe abdominal pain
- chest pain, cough, shortness of breath
- severe headache, dizziness, weakness, or numbness
- blurred vision
- yellowing of the skin

Contraception 911

With so much at stake, why don't doctors make their patients aware of emergency birth control methods during routine physical exams? That's what a lot of reproductive health experts have been asking. The result is a full-fledged campaign to increase awareness of morning-after contraception among women and doctors. For detailed information about "morning-after" contraception:

- Call the Emergency Contraception Hotline (800-584-9911), which describes the options and will put you in touch with local providers who can prescribe them.
- Read *Emergency Contraception: The Nation's Best Kept Secret* (Bridging the Gap Communications, $12.95, 800-847-3988).
- Visit the Emergency Contraception Web site: http://opr.princeton.edu/ec/ec.html.

A Word About the Abortion Pill

As this book went to press, the FDA was considering the approval of the drug mifepristone, known in France as RU-486. An advisory com-

EMERGENCY CONTRACEPTION METHODS			
Method	Can Be Used Up to . . .	Effectiveness	Cautions
Combined Oral Contraceptives	72 hours after inter-course, followed by a second dose 12 hours later	75%	Often causes nausea and vomiting; should not be used by women with a history of heart disease, stroke, migraine, or cancer.
Mini-pills	48 hours after inter-course, followed by a second dose 12 hours later	75%	An alternative for women who can't take estrogen; less likely to cause nausea.
Copper IUD	Seven days after intercourse	99%	The IUD is not recommended for women at risk for sexually transmitted diseases.

mittee has already concluded that the controversial French abortion pill is safe and effective. The Population Council, a nonprofit organization, holds the patent rights to mifepristone. It conducted studies on the drug in seventeen sites around the country involving 2,100 women. This data forms the basis of the Council's application to the FDA.

Abortion with mifepristone involves a two-step procedure: Women go to a physician's office or clinic and take several mifepristone tablets, which interrupt the pregnancy. Two days later they return to the office for a dose of another drug, a prostaglandin (called misoprostol), which triggers uterine contractions that expel the fetus. Women typically experience cramping and bleeding—sometimes heavy. Many of the women in the studies reported that taking the abortion pill gave them a sense of control over the process, that it was less invasive, and that it seemed more natural than a surgical abortion.

A similar abortion regimen involves the drug methotrexate, which is currently available and approved for other medical uses, including: severe rheumatoid arthritis, lupus, and Crohn's disease. The process works the same way as mifepristone but takes longer. The patient returns to the clinic for misoprostol, the prostaglandin, a week later. Methotrexate is not quite as effective as mifepristone, and some women require a second prostaglandin dose. Both drugs are appropriate for use in ending pregnancies up to about ten weeks.

When you are ready to become pregnant there are several things you can do to make sure you have a healthy pregnancy. According to the American Medical Association and the American College of Obstetricians and Gynecologists, you should:

✓ Schedule an appointment with your provider several months before you intend to get pregnant. In addition to the general workup, you should be tested for several conditions that can harm your fetus: toxoplasmosis, rubella, hepatitis B. If you have other health conditions that make pregnancy risky—such as diabetes or high blood pressure—this is the time to find out how to best manage them.

✓ If there is a possibility you could have a sexually transmitted disease, ask to be tested. Some STDs can have serious health consequences for your baby or may complicate the pregnancy. If

Who Should Pay for Contraception?

At present, fewer than 20 percent of large group health insurance plans and 40 percent of HMOs cover reversible forms of birth control, according to the Alan Guttmacher Institute. That means women themselves must pick up the tab for contraception.

Legislation proposed in the Senate in early 1998, called the Equity in Prescription Insurance and Contraceptive Coverage Act (EPICC), would require insurance companies that cover prescription drugs and devices to include FDA-approved prescription contraceptives. According to the bill's proponents, when insurers treat contraceptives differently from other prescription drugs, they send a message that they are willing to cover all of men's prescription drug needs but not women's. The expense for covering contraceptive needs is minimal, however—about $1.25 per woman per month, according to the National Family Planning and Reproductive Health Association.

At the time this book went to press, the bill was expected to pass.

Conscious Conception

With all the time, money, and psychic energy spent on preventing pregnancy, it is often astonishing to women who are ready for childbearing when they fail to conceive immediately.

In desperation, couples often turn to fertility clinics. The desire for a baby turns into a financial and emotional nightmare for some. Fertility clinics, which have exploded in number during the last two decades, are often guilty of subjecting couples to unimaginable stress as they attempt one high-tech method after another with no success. In fact, the Federal Trade Commission has begun to crack down on clinics that exaggerate their success rates.

Barring a genuine organic problem (with either partner) or illness, many fertility problems often boil down to simple timing. The beauty of fertility awareness as birth control is that its principles and practices can be used as tools for triggering pregnancy.

Knowledge of your reproductive physiology can also be useful in detecting pregnancy once it has occurred and to detect impaired fertility. Toni Weschler, M.P.H., believes many diagnostic tests for infertility are ill-timed or altogether unnecessary. Charting your fertility signs can help you work with your doctor to narrow the range of problems.

If you are using basal body temperature as a measure of fertility, note that a postovulatory temperature rise that's sustained for eighteen or more days is a sign of pregnancy. Conversely, a relatively steady basal body temperature may reveal a lack of ovulation and can also alert a woman to a fertility problem.

Things that can hinder conception:

- Low percentage of body fat (less than 18 percent).
- Use of lubricants, which alter the cervical mucus and impede the movement of sperm.
- Either parents' use of drugs, including antihistamines, caffeine, nicotine, alcohol, and marijuana.
- Excessive stress.
- Heat (hot tubs and saunas kill sperm).
- Either parents' exposure to toxic substances, such as lead.

If you are unable to become pregnant after a year of unprotected sexual intercourse, you may have a fertility problem. If you reach the one-year mark, talk to your health-care provider about the options available to you for identifying and correcting the problem. (If you are over thirty, however, you may want to seek help sooner.)

Workplace Reproductive Hazards

Some occupations involve workplace hazards that put potential parents at risk for having children with birth defects and other problems. These jobs include those that require employees to work with toxic chemicals and even those that expose you to some common office equipment, such as video display terminals. If you are concerned about workplace hazards, the following organizations can provide information:

- The Coalition of Labor Union Women, Reproductive Rights Project, 1126 Sixteenth Street NW, Washington, DC 20036; 202-466-4610.
- 9 to 5, National Association of Working Women, 614 Superior Avenue, NW, Suite 852, Cleveland, OH 44113. Job Survival Hotline: 800-522-0925.
- MASSCOSH, 555 Amory Street, Boston, MA 02130; 617-524-6686. (Publishes the guide *Confronting Reproductive Health Hazards on the Job.*)

The Facts of Fertilization

Out of the hundreds of millions of sperm that travel into the female reproductive system (specifically to the fallopian tubes) during sexual in-

you are HIV-positive, you can take steps to minimize the risk of transmitting the virus to your unborn child. (See "AIDS and Pregnancy," page 174.)

✓ If you are adopted and know little about your birth parents, or have a family history of a genetic disorder, ask to be referred to a genetic counselor, who can evaluate your risk of having a child with a birth defect.

✓ At least three months before you plan to conceive, begin taking a daily vitamin supplement containing 400 micrograms of folic acid, which has been shown to reduce the risk of certain birth defects.

✓ Start a fitness program. Exercising during pregnancy is good for you and your baby and may help to ease childbirth.

✓ Do not drink alcohol, or take over-the-counter drugs. If you take prescription drugs for any health condition, discuss the potential risks with your doctor.

✓ Quit smoking. Smoking is not only bad for your baby, it may also diminish your fertility. And studies show that smokers have higher miscarriage rates.

✓ If you have ever been pregnant and had a problem such as miscarriage, premature delivery, or abnormal fetal development, you will want to discuss the possibility of a recurrence with your provider.

✓ If you have been on oral contraceptives, switch to a barrier method of birth control at least three months before trying to conceive. If you are using an IUD, you should have it removed a month or so before conceiving and use a barrier method in the interim.

✓ Raise any age-related concerns with your provider. Specifically you may want to inquire about difficulty in conceiving; your risk for having a miscarriage, stillbirth, or low-birth-weight baby; and the incidence of birth defects and chromosomal abnormalities.

tercourse, several eventually try to penetrate the egg. Only one actually enters it. Once this superior sperm has made it to the center, the sperm and egg merge. The resulting one-cell embryo is called a *zygote*.

Within twelve hours, the new cell has already divided into two cells. In another twelve hours these two cells will have divided yet again. And the process continues, all of the cells doubling every twelve hours.

During the next four or five days, the egg makes its way to the uterus, where it will grow for approximately 260 days. Now the egg is a cluster of cells grouped around a fluid-filled cavity, called the *blastocyst*. Part of the *blastocyst* will produce the embryo. The outer cell layer, called the *trophoblast*, becomes the placenta, which will nourish the growing fetus.

Meanwhile, the ovaries have been secreting the hormone progesterone, which helps build up the uterine lining, making implantation possible. After clinging to the lining for several days, the egg begins to produce an enzyme that allows it to firmly attach to the lining, where it will be nourished by the mother's blood. By Day 12 after fertilization, the egg is firmly entrenched within the uterus.

At this point a woman is officially pregnant, even though she has not missed a period or even experienced any pregnancy symptoms. Miscarriage is common in the early days after fertilization; indeed, as many as half of all fertilizations end in miscarriage.

The egg and sperm have each brought twenty-three chromosomes containing thousands of genes to the union for a total of forty-six chromosomes. These genes determine the gender and all the physical characteristics of the new individual—from eye and skin color to intelligence and creativity.

Conception Clues

Getting pregnant is a significant event to be sure, but you may not feel momentous changes right away. The first clue that you have conceived may simply be a missed or scanty period. Many women experience breast tenderness and pain or especially sensitive nipples.

Morning sickness (a misnomer, since it can strike at any time of day) may begin as early as a few days after a missed period. Common in the first trimester of pregnancy, it is characterized by nausea, queasiness, or vomiting, and may range from mild to extreme.

Frequent urination afflicts many women, due to hormonal changes and, later, to the pressure of the developing fetus on the bladder. You may also feel overcome with fatigue in the early days of pregnancy.

If you experience any of these symptoms and have missed a period, it's a good idea to get a pregnancy test. The sooner you know for certain that you are pregnant, the better prepared you will be to make sound decisions about your care.

Home Pregnancy Tests

So you think you're pregnant? The earliest way to know for sure is to have a pregnancy test. You can do this at a doctor's office or at home with an over-the-counter pregnancy test.

By Day 4 after fertilization, the egg begins to secrete a hormone called human chorionic gonadotropin (hCG), which can be detected in blood or urine. Today most tests are done with urine because it can be obtained easily. These tests detect the presence of hCG and depend on a reaction between hCG and hCG antibodies. A second reaction reveals whether the first reaction has taken place—often by changing color.

Home pregnancy tests contain a solution that's mixed with urine in a test tube. After a period of time (from a few minutes to two hours depending on the test), a dark ring forms or the color changes if you are pregnant. It's best to take the test first thing in the morning to get the best urine sample.

Accuracy depends on many factors, including collecting the urine according to package instructions. Follow these instructions carefully and keep in mind that sometimes very early pregnancies will not show up because the levels of hCG are not as high then as they will be further into the pregnancy. It's important to wait at least until Day 28 of your cycle. If you have a positive result, see your doctor or other health-care provider to confirm your test and begin prenatal care.

Fast-Track Fertility

You and your partner have made one of the biggest decisions you will ever face: to have a baby. But even the strongest desire for a child, as many discouraged couples discover, does not mean conception will happen right away. Researchers have recently shed a brighter light on the process, which can help you make the most of your efforts. Here are some common babymaking myths and realities:

Rumor: Pregnancy can occur anywhere from several days before ovulation to several days after.

Reality: According to a 1995 study from the National Institute of Environmental Health Sciences, women's fertile period lasts six days—the five days before ovulation and the day of ovulation itself—and then stops abruptly. Although it is possible to get pregnant by having sex five days before ovulation, the chances of conceiving are greatest when intercourse occurs closer to ovulation. You can identify when you're ovulating by watching for the physical changes involved in fertility awareness (cervical mucus becoming sticky and stretchy or body temperature rising slightly) or by using an ovulation predictor kit.

Rumor: *Men should abstain from sex several days before their partner's ovulation in order to build up their sperm count.*

Reality: Under ordinary circumstances, there's plenty of sperm to achieve pregnancy. In fact, frequent sex is optimal. Couples who have sex every day during the fertile times have a 25 percent chance of conceiving in any given cycle; those who make love every other day have a 22 percent chance. By comparison, couples who have intercourse just once a week have only a 10 percent chance of conceiving, according to the National Institute of Environmental Health Sciences study. (Men with low sperm counts, however, may be advised to have intercourse every other day, so as to allow time to build up their sperm levels.)

Rumor: *A woman's orgasm has nothing to do with conception.*

Reality: According to British researchers, female orgasm appears to facilitate conception, probably by drawing ejaculate into the upper reproductive tract.

Rumor: *Men should wear boxers, not briefs, to promote conception.*

Reality: A 1997 study found that wearing close-fitting underwear did not lower sperm counts.

Are You Ovulating?

If you're ready to get pregnant, you don't want to waste a minute. One way of upping the odds is to use an over-the-counter ovulation prediction kit. Available at pharmacies, ovulation predictors can help you pinpoint ovulation, the time when you are most fertile. They work by detecting luteinizing hormone (LH), a chemical that triggers the release of an egg from one of your ovaries. This surge of LH usually happens midcycle.

The tests can be tricky to use and interpret, so it's important to follow the package directions exactly. They work best when you have a regular cycle. If your cycle is irregular, you will need to track the length of your cycle over a period of several months and determine the average cycle length. Then you take a urine sample, usually in the middle part of the day, for five days or so. When the test detects an increase in LH you will likely ovulate within the next twenty-four to forty-eight hours. Be aware that you may not ovulate every cycle, especially if you are under stress.

Warning: Using the test to *prevent* pregnancy is risky, as sperm can live in the female reproductive tract for several days; by the time you detect ovulation, there still may be time for a sperm to fertilize the newly released egg.

The Future of Contraception

The perfect contraception would be noninvasive, easy to use, convenient, and foolproof. It would not contain unnatural levels of chemicals, pose health risks, have side effects, or interfere with lovemaking. It would be inexpensive and reversible.

Unfortunately there is no such thing as perfect contraception. And our birth control choices are unlikely to broaden significantly anytime soon.

Even as many scientists herald a contraceptive revolution in the lab, the climate for bringing new wares to market is gloomy. To start with, it takes a minimum of fifteen years to develop and market a new pharmaceutical from start to finish, and it can cost between $20 and $70 million to get the drug or device to market, according to the Planned Parenthood Federation. Political and legal issues also stand in the way of giving American women new contraceptive options. In fact, women in other countries often have access to a greater number of birth control choices than their U.S. counterparts.

Still, the work of scientists worldwide in this area is intriguing. Many aim to improve upon available methods; others strike out in bold new directions—such as contraceptives for men. Some researchers even predict that gene therapy could be used to control fertility sometime in the distant future. As of this writing there are several contraceptives new to the market or expected to soon enter it:

Polyurethane condoms are particularly useful for people who are allergic to latex. There are several variations, including one so-called bidonnable condom, which can be used on either side. That means it can be rolled on even in the dark.

Lea's Shield is an ingenious one-size-fits-all diaphragm made of silicone. It contains a special one-way valve that provides suction so that it fits more snugly over the cervix. The valve also allows cervical secretions to escape. A small "handle" facilitates easy removal. It can be held in place for forty-eight hours.

Femcap, a new cervical cap made of silicone rubber.

Mirena, a new IUD, releases estrogen and progestin over a five-year period, thus combining the best features of hormonal contraception (superior effectiveness and numerous health benefits) and the IUD (long-lasting protection) for women who can use it. Currently available in fourteen Europe and Asian countries, the IUD was expected to reach the U.S. market during 1998 or 1999.

For Women

High-Tech Fertility Awareness

In Britain, women currently have access to a new birth control device called Persona, which makes use of a computerized hormone monitor and urine test sticks. A woman uses a test stick eight times a month to measure levels of two hormones in the morning urine. The monitor takes a reading from the stick and uses information previously programmed into the computer about the woman's cycle to determine whether she is ovulating. The device then either gives her a green, red, or yellow light to indicate whether sex is safe. (Yellow means more information is needed.) Manufacturers claim Persona has an effectiveness rate of 95 percent, although it is not a good form of birth control for women with very irregular cycles (less than twenty-three days or more than thirty-five). Persona is in clinical trials in the United States.

A Better Pill

It's good; let's make it better, say pharmaceutical companies. They are tinkering with the estrogen and progestin dosage so as to reduce the dose while maintaining the method's effectiveness, trying new estrogens that would reduce current side effects, such as mood swings and weight gain, and developing new progestins to alleviate other side effects, such as acne and facial hair growth.

Melatonin

This hormone, which is responsible for seasonal breeding cycles in many mammalian species, has been found to shut off the brain centers that direct ovulation. When combined with progesterone in a pill, melatonin appears to effectively suppress fertility in humans. So far, the pill has been tested in the Netherlands with good results.

New Implant Systems

Like Norplant, these systems, which go under the names Implanon, Uniplant, and Nesterone, are in various stages of development. They're intended to reduce the number of capsules used and vary the time length of effectiveness. Some are biodegradable, which eliminates the problems of removal.

Vaginal Rings

These donut-shaped rings fit in the vagina and release either progestin alone or a combination of estrogen and progestin. Though they do not last as long as implants, they offer considerable convenience over taking a daily pill and are under the immediate control of the user—an important feature for many women. Expected availability: the year 2000.

New Injectables

New hormonal contraceptive injections are similar to Depo-Provera but last longer.

Better Barrier Methods

The Today Sponge was removed from the market in 1995 due to concerns about manufacturing practices. However, a new sponge, called Protectaid, is in development. It combines three types of chemicals that kill both sperm and disease-promoting microbes. In lab studies it inactivated HIV as well as chlamydia and trichomoniasis, two major bacterial diseases.

Also on the drawing board: disposable diaphragms with a spermicide already applied and better spermicides that don't irritate vaginal walls—as some now do (especially those that contain nonoxynol-9)—and that also protect against disease.

Mifepristone (RU-486)

In addition to its use as a nonsurgical abortion drug, mifepristone could play a much less controversial role as a means of contraception. Scottish researchers have already explored its use as an alternative method of emergency contraception. It was more effective than the current methods (specific doses of traditional oral contraceptives) and caused fewer side effects.

Mifepristone could also be taken in a continuous low dose to prevent ovulation or as a once-a-month contraception. Researchers in Sweden see it working this way: A woman would use a home fertility kit to detect ovulation (the test kits detect a sudden rise in luteinizing hormone, which signals the release of a mature egg from the ovary). Then she would take a dose of mifepristone to prevent pregnancy.

For Men

Yes, ladies, you heard right—a *male* contraceptive. The challenge: to stop the constant production of millions of sperm without diminishing sex drive and function. Remember, female contraception only has to stop the action of a single egg a month. Researchers must also find a mechanism of delivery that provides more than a week's worth of protection.

Testosterone Injections

Weekly hormone injections reduce the concentration of sperm in semen to either very low or undetectable levels. A two-year, four-continent clinical trial has shown the method to be 98.6 percent effective. The prospects for approval are good—it's safe and very effective, but getting men to submit to weekly shots could be a challenge.

Mechanical Interventions

A nontoxic substance is injected into the vas deferens (the duct carrying sperm from the testicles), forming a plug that blocks the passage of sperm. If a man wishes to restore his fertility later, his doctor can inject a second substance to dissolve the plug. Developed in India, the process is in clinical trials with humans.

Implant System

This one-year contraceptive implant suppresses sperm production while maintaining sex drive. The U.S.–based Population Council, a non-profit organization, has started human trials but is years away from a marketable method. In 1998 trials to determine its safety were under way.

Plant Compounds

The best known, called gossypol, is derived from cottonseed oil and has been studied for two decades. Though it effectively suppresses sperm, it also causes irreversible infertility in some men. *Tripterygium wilfordii*, a vine that grows in southern China, has also shown promise as an effective male contraceptive, but is a long way from human trials. Many kinks must be worked out before either substance is a viable contraceptive alternative. However, they may ultimately offer the advantage of having fewer sexual side effects.

Antifertility Vaccines

Chemicals neutralize the hormones required for sperm production or maturation. One of the vaccine's side effects is the suppression of sex drive, so the vaccine would have to be combined with an implant that supplies the hormones responsible for libido. In 1998 the Population Council had begun early-stage trials to determine its safety and effectiveness. Only a few men have been "immunized" so far, but the research is progressing.

Contraceptive, Fertility, and Pregnancy Resources

Organizations

Planned Parenthood Federation of America Inc.
810 Seventh Avenue
New York, NY 10019
800-230-PLAN
There are more than 900 Planned Parenthood Clinics in America. They offer reproductive health care and education.

The Norplant Foundation
703-706-5933
A nonprofit organization that provides information on the Norplant implant system.

AVSC, International
79 Madison Avenue
New York, NY 10016
212-561-8000
Access to Voluntary and Safe Contraception provides information on family planning and reproduction, especially voluntary sterilization.

Cervical Cap Ltd.
430 Monterey Avenue, Suite 1B
Los Gatos, CA 95030
408-395-2100
Information about cervical caps and finding providers who can prescribe them.

Billings Ovulation Method
Natural Family Planning Center of Washington, D.C.
8514 Bradmoor Drive
Bethesda, MD 20817-3810
301-897-9323 or 800-484-7416 (code #1001)
Offers information on this fertility awareness method of birth control.

Northwest Family Services
4805 N.E. Glisan
Portland, OR 97213
503-215-6377
A resource on fertility awareness.

Fertility Awareness Network
Barbara Feldman, Coordinator
P.O. Box 1190
New York, NY 10009
A resource on fertility awareness. (Send SASE plus $4 for an information packet.)

Fertility Awareness Services
Suzannah Cooper Doyle
P.O. Box 986
Corvallis, OR 97339
A resource on fertility awareness. (Send SASE with 55¢ postage for information.)

American Board of Medical Genetics
9650 Rockville Pike
Bethesda, MD 20814
301-571-1825
Provides information about genetics counseling.

National Society of Genetic Counselors
233 Canterbury Drive
Wallingford, PA 19086
215-872-7608
Provides referrals to genetics counseling training programs.

National Maternal and Child Health Clearinghouse
38th and R Streets, NW
Washington, DC 20057
202-625-8410
Offers general reproductive health information.

March of Dimes Birth Defects Foundation
1275 Mamaroneck Avenue
White Plains, NY 10605
914-428-7100
Offers information on birth-defect prevention and research.

RESOLVE, Inc.
1310 Broadway
Somerville, MA 02144-1731
617-623-1156
Provides information on infertility.

Books

The Birth Control Book, by Samuel A. Pasquale, M.D., and Jennifer Cadoff (Ballantine Books, 1996).

Taking Charge of Your Fertility, by Toni Weschler, M.P.H. (HarperPerennial, 1996).

Protecting Your Baby-to-Be: Preventing Birth Defects in the First Trimester, by Margie Profet (Addison-Wesley Publishing Company, 1995).

Before You Conceive: The Complete Prepregnancy Guide, by John R. Sussman, M.D. and B. Blake Levitt (Bantam Books, 1989).

Conception, Pregnancy and Birth, by Miriam Stoppard, M.D. (Dorling Kindersley Publishing, 1993).

Mayo Clinic Complete Book of Pregnancy and Baby's First Year (William Morrow Company, Inc., 1994).

What to Expect When You're Expecting, by Arlene Eisenberg, Heidi E. Markoff, and Sandee E. Hathaway, B.S.N. (Workman Publishing Company, Inc., 1986).

5 | Sexual Wisdom

In our culture, most sex education programs limit discussion of human reproduction to the mechanical details of sexual intercourse. They tend to ignore the
emotional and pleasurable dimensions that give sexuality its meaning and significance—not to mention other forms of sexual expression.

This sexual schism is not just limiting, it is harmful. You can't talk about sexual intercourse without talking about penises, after all, but many girls grow up
not even knowing that they have a sexual organ known as the clitoris. These girls
grow up not knowing that they have a right to feel good about sex and to seek
the pleasure that intimacy has to offer. They end up literally groping in the dark
for information—and affirmation—about their sexuality. This legacy follows
them into adulthood, shaping their self-image and the quality of their relationships.

If your own sex education started so inauspiciously, you owe yourself an adult
education course focused on the pleasure principles of sex. This chapter starts
with the premise that fulfilling your sexual potential is a basic component of sexual health. Sexual health encompasses knowing what turns you on and learning
how to get your sexual needs met, just as it involves understanding how to obtain the best Pap smear, choosing the right birth control method, and knowing
how to protect yourself from sexually transmitted diseases.

The pages that follow are intended to enlighten you about how your body is
designed for pleasure and to explore the ways that you can seek and achieve sexual satisfaction. As you become more knowledgeable, you will find yourself in a
better position to take responsibility for your sexual pleasure and communicate
your needs to your partner—one of the foundations of healthy sexuality.

Sex Surveys

Sex surveys fill a void in a culture such as ours where people don't talk openly
about sexual behaviors. They purport to tell us what other people are doing in
bed and when and how often they do it.

How accurately do surveys represent sexual behavior? It's a good question.

People are not always truthful when revealing information about their intimate lives. They may tell the interviewer what they expect him to hear or what they think is socially acceptable. Even Alfred Kinsey, the zoologist-turned-sexologist who conducted the groundbreaking studies on sexual conduct in the 1940s and 50s, relied on the self-reports of people who volunteered the details of their sex lives rather than a representative sampling of all Americans.

The sweeping "Sex in America" study, released by the University of Chicago in 1994, is today's best guess as to what's going on in bedrooms across the country. The researchers interviewed more than 3,000 randomly selected men and women to arrive at their data and achieved an impressive 79 percent response rate. (By contrast, the Hite Report of the 1970s had a mere 3 percent.) In scientific terms, it was a well designed and rigorous survey.

The data paints a portrait of a far more sexually conservative society than one would imagine based on how our media depict Americans' sex lives. The survey showed that we have less sex with fewer partners and engage in fewer exotic practices than soap operas and daytime talk shows might suggest. For example, 80 percent of Americans reported having one or fewer sexual partners in the year prior to the survey interview.

Some other survey highlights:

- On average, Americans have sex about once a week.
- The median number of sexual partners over a lifetime for men is six; for women, two.
- Some 75 percent of married men and 85 percent of married women are faithful to their spouses.
- Of those surveyed, 1.4 percent of women and 2.8 percent of men identify themselves as homosexual.
- After vaginal intercourse (and before giving and receiving oral sex), the most popular form of sex was "watching my partner undress."
- Some 25 percent of Americans have had anal sex.
- By and large, we choose partners who are very much like ourselves in terms of race, income, and education. In general, the researchers found, opposites do not attract.

One of the survey's most troubling statistics related to sexual coercion—22 percent of women reported having been forced to do something sexually that they didn't want to. Women who reported having been touched sexually as children were more likely as adults to say they had experienced painful sex, anxiety about sexual performance, and/or emotional problems that interfered with intimacy. This alarming data speaks to the long-term repercussions of childhood sexual abuse and our society's poor record in dealing with the issues of abuse and forced sex.

The "Sex in America" survey has limitations. Despite the researchers' best intentions, it's likely that some respondents lied about their sexual behavior. For instance, among respondents who were interviewed when they were alone, some 17 percent admitted to having sex with two or more partners in the previous year. The figure dropped to five percent among respondents who were apparently within earshot of a spouse or other sexual partner.

Remember that even the best sex surveys are inherently limited. So don't worry if your own sexuality falls short of the standards set by *Melrose Place,* or that your bedroom behavior might be considered abnormal. What's important is accepting your own sexual feelings and desires—even when they seem to conflict with societal norms and sexual "correctness."

The Enigmatic "O"

Learning what turns you on and how to reach your orgasmic potential is a basic, and often ignored, human need. As you come to know more about your sexuality, you can achieve greater comfort and healthiness in your relationships.

The first step is understanding what's involved in sexual response. Much of what we know about this aspect of sexuality comes from the pioneering work of William Masters, M.D., and Virginia Johnson, the famed sex research team. Masters and Johnson identified the four distinct stages of sexual response—excitement, plateau, orgasm, and resolution—each marked by changes in blood flow.

Sexuality, they discovered, is a genuine body-mind experience. Sexual response starts in the mind. All kinds of stimuli can trigger sexual feelings—the sight or smell of a partner or touch itself. Once arousal begins, the brain sends the biochemical signals that initiate the physical responses leading to sexual plateau. As this happens, blood rushes into the genitals. In men, the erectile tissue in the penis fills with blood, causing it to expand in length and width. The penis becomes rigid enough to penetrate the vagina. The testicles become engorged with blood and draw up closer to the body. The nipples may harden.

Women experience similar changes, although they are not as obvious. The genital structures become engorged with blood, and the erectile tissue of the clitoris becomes hard. The labia turn red or purple, and the vagina becomes moist with natural lubrication. The vagina literally tips up in preparation for intercourse. The nipples become erect and may even darken, and the breasts swell. At the end of the plateau phase, the clitoris becomes hidden beneath the clitoral hood. Some 75 percent of women experience a sexual "flush" or red rash on the skin.

During orgasm, both men and women experience a contraction of the rectal sphincter, a reduction in voluntary muscle control, and involuntary and rhythmic muscle spasms in the pelvic area. In men, the contractions serve to draw fluids and sperm into the urethra and then expel them outside the body. Women may also ejaculate fluid during orgasm.

Both genders experience a deep relaxation as the body's systems return to the normal, unaroused state. This process is faster in men; in women it can take half an hour. The objective experience of orgasm in men and women seems to be similar. When people were asked to write down what orgasm felt like, researchers couldn't tell if the author was a man or a woman.

There are some important differences between the ways men and women achieve orgasm, however. Men tend to be more visually oriented and more easily aroused in general. After all, an erection is an unparalleled feedback mechanism; it lets men know beyond a doubt that they are aroused, and this can itself feed sexual excitement, says Eileen M. Palace, Ph.D., of Tulane University in New Orleans. Conversely, some women aren't aware when they are sexually excited. This may be one of the reasons they often take longer to reach orgasm.

Women do have some distinct advantages, though: Men usually require some downtime before a second orgasm is possible. This so-called refractory period gets longer with age. Not so, women. Some can respond immediately to additional stimulation and have more orgasms.

Although every woman responds differently during sex, women can call on a multitude of strategies to reach orgasm. Some women experience orgasm through stimulation of their nipples alone or even by nothing more than thinking sexy thoughts. Many respond to stimulation of sensitive tissue within the vagina. About 40 percent of women experience nocturnal orgasms—spontaneous orgasms that occur during sleep, akin to men's wet dreams. Some women are multiorgasmic, while others enjoy only one powerful climax.

Women and Orgasm: Just the Facts

- Some 60 percent of women discovered orgasm on their own.
- Less than 50 percent have had orgasms through intercourse.
- Fully 70 percent have masturbated to orgasm.
- By age fifteen, 23 percent have had their first orgasm.
- Up to 70 percent have faked orgasm.
- Sixty-four percent have had "no-touch" orgasms induced by fantasy or imagery.
- Forty percent have nocturnal orgasms.
- Ten to 12 percent have never had an orgasm.
- Average length of time women need to reach orgasm: eight minutes (the range: one minute to half an hour).
- Orgasm itself generally lasts from seven to more than one hundred seconds.

Source: The Kinsey Institute for Research in Sex, Gender and Reproduction

The C-Spot

If you thought that female sexuality centered on the pea-shaped organ known as the clitoris, you are right—and wrong. It turns out that the tiny pink bulb that you see when you pull back the clitoris's protective hood is just the end of a complex internal structure. The clitoris has distinct parts in addition to the glans and hood: two long clitoral "legs" (also called crura); erectile tissue, including the urethral sponge and perineal sponge; muscles; nerve endings; and an intricate network of blood vessels. A spongy mass of tissue envelops the pelvic area. When the clitoris is stimulated, this tissue becomes engorged and swells significantly.

Like the vagina, the clitoris and its underlying structure have been virtually ignored in medical and scientific research. Medical texts give no hint to the complexity and size of its extensive infrastructure. No wonder women are often confused about what they find stimulating in bed.

In 1980, the Federation of Feminist Women's Health Centers set out to remedy the oversight and let women in on the mystery of this sexual organ. Using the scant bit of information available and their own observations, they wrote and published *A New View of a Woman's Body*. This

A Cross Section of the Nonerect Clitoris

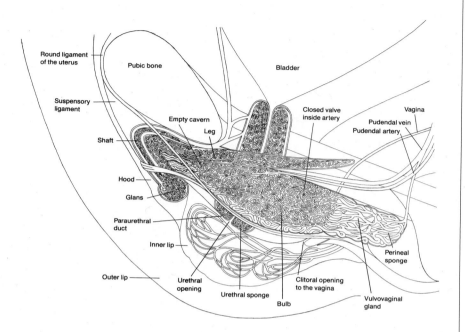

The clitoris, greatly magnified, in its nonerect state. The intricate maze, created by the blood vessels and capillaries in the tissues of the glans, shaft, and legs, is called the corpus cavernosum, which literally means body of caverns. The urethral sponge, perineal sponge, and bulbs differ from corpus cavernosum in that they are made up of tissue that is more elastic and does not become as hard during erection. This tissue is called corpus spongiosum. In the nonerect state, the valves of the veins are open.

book described and illustrated the remarkable clitoral structure in all its glory. The authors observed that the clitoris is very similar to the penis and related male organs—most of it is simply hidden from view. Moreover, since the clitoris appears to be more extensive than previously believed, making distinctions between clitoral and vaginal orgasms may be moot. The nerve-rich urethral sponge is located alongside the vagina, so orgasmic response from intercourse is essentially linked to the clitoris, anyway.

A Cross Section of the Clitoris During Sexual Arousal

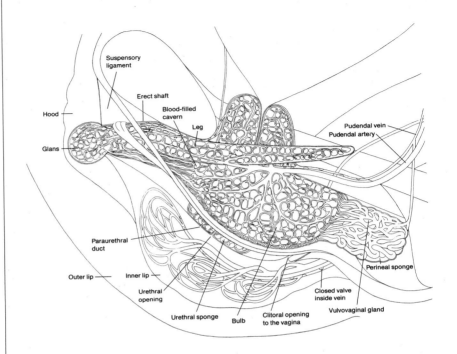

During sexual arousal, the intricate chambers of these tissues fill with blood, which is then trapped by valves, and the entire clitoris enlarges and changes dramatically. The glans and shaft become erect and maintain their positions until resolution. Underneath, the muscles are taut and contract in response to sexual stimulation.

Illustrations: *A New View of a Woman's Body,* Federation of Feminist Health Centers © 1991 by Suzann Gage, L. Ac., R.N.C., N.P.

Whether or not you believe that vaginal orgasms are different from the clitoral type—a point of continuing debate—viewing the illustrations in *A New View of a Woman's Body* is a revelation. Seeing that the glans of the clitoris is literally the tip of the iceberg could help explain why a woman might feel unsatisfied if stimulation were confined to it, why direct stimulation of the glans is unnecessary for orgasm, or for that matter why so much seems to be going on when women are sexually excited.

The bottom line: Understanding and visualizing the source of pleasurable sensations is part of realizing your sexual potential.

To order a copy of A New View of a Woman's Body, *write: Feminist Health Press, 8240 Santa Monica Boulevard, Los Angeles, CA 90046; 213-650-1508. (Include $19.95, plus $4 shipping and handling.)*

Orgasm Origins

Some 70 percent of women require direct clitoral stimulation to climax. But many experts now believe that there are other routes to orgasm.

This is a reversal of the common belief held since the research of Alfred Kinsey changed America's ideas about sexuality in the 1950s. One of the main tenets of his findings was that the clitoris is the sole source of female pleasure, and the vagina itself is devoid of nerve endings. Masters and Johnson also accepted this point of view.

In the 1980s, researchers John Perry, Ph.D., and Beverly Whipple, Ph.D., promoted the G-spot, named for the German-born gynecologist Ernst Grafenberg who first identified it in the 1950s. The G-spot is a bean-sized area that can be felt through the vaginal wall about halfway between the back of the pubic bone and the cervix. It feels like a small lump but swells when stimulated and, according to Whipple, eventually produces an unusually intense orgasm.

The idea that the vagina is sensitive to stimulation and capable of triggering pleasurable feelings is now fairly well accepted. In fact, researchers have identified other areas of special sensitivity in the vagina, including the cervix itself (*see "The New Sexual Geography," page 99*).

Some experts believe that vaginal orgasms are distinctly different from clitorally based orgasms:

Clitoral Orgasms Masters and Johnson coined the term "tenting" to describe the physical changes accompanying clitoral orgasm: The internal pelvic organs are pulled up toward the breast, and the top part of the vagina balloons, says Whipple. The sensation is a twinge of exquisitely intense pleasure.

Vaginal Orgasms During vaginal orgasms, the opposite appears to occur: The internal organs are pushed downward, and the upper vagina contracts. Many women report a diffused, warm, or melting pleasure.

Female Ejaculation

Many women report expelling a fluid during orgasm, especially when the G-spot is stimulated. This fluid has been described as looking like watered-down skim milk. Some researchers and medical providers dispute the evidence for female ejaculation or suggest the fluid is actually urine. However, since the early 1980s, researchers have published some thirty studies documenting the occurrence of female ejaculation or analyzed its composition. The fluid, called prostatic acid phosphatase, is basically made up of sugars (glucose and fructose).

If the experts can't agree on female ejaculation, it's not surprising that many women are confused or embarrassed about this aspect of their sexuality. According to Whipple, some women have even had corrective surgery because they thought they were incontinent. In studies, other women have reported holding back orgasm for fear of releasing this fluid.

Female ejaculation appears to be a perfectly normal part of the sexual process. Some researchers believe it may even signify particularly intense arousal.

How to Find Your G-Spot

The G-Spot can be a little difficult to locate at first, but it's worth the effort. Beverly Whipple, Ph.D., who helped let the world in on this mysterious source of feminine erotic pleasure, offers this advice for finding it:

"The problem with trying to locate the Grafenberg spot by yourself is that you need very long fingers and/or a very short vagina to reach the area while lying on your back.

"A few women have reported that they are able to locate their G-spot by themselves while seated on a toilet. After emptying their bladders they explore along the anterior (upper front) wall of the vagina with a firm pressure pushing up toward the navel. Some women find it helpful to apply a downward pressure on the abdomen with their other hand, just above the pubic bone on top of the pubic hair line. As the G-spot is stimulated and begins to swell, it can often be felt between the two sets of fingers.

"It often feels like a small spongy bean and in some women swells to the size of a half dollar. Experiment with the Grafenberg spot. You will need to use a heavier pressure than you do on the clitoris, and you may feel the sensations deeper inside than you do with clitoral stimulation."

After you have discovered the spot on your own, you can share your experience with a partner. The best position for stimulating it during intercourse is with the woman sitting on top of the man or through rear vaginal entry. Don't worry if you can't find it at first. Think of G-spot stimulation as just one of many sexual options, Whipple suggests.

The New Sexual Geography

Just when you were getting around to finding your G-spot, sex researchers have identified "new" female erogenous zones (*see below*).

The anterior fornix erogenous (or AFE) zone was recently identified by a gynecologist in Malaysia. Called the A-spot, the zone appears to increase lubrication, making sex more comfortable. Like the G-spot, this

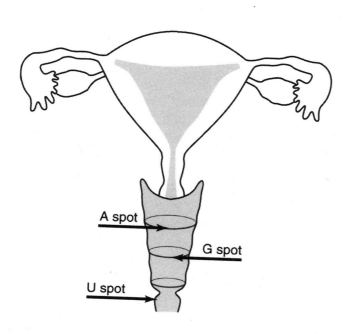

Robin Michals, 1998

zone can be found on the upper vaginal wall, although it is closer to the cervix.

Also on the sexual geography map is an area of the urethral canal called the U-spot, which offers yet another source of sexual feeling. It can be found nearer to the vaginal opening.

Experts say these sexy spots can increase your sexual options, but it is important to remember that they are not essential for bliss in bed. According to Whipple, "Any place on the body can produce erotic sensations." Three quarters of women and 61 percent of men in a recent survey reported the neck to be an important erogenous zone. Nine percent of women and eight percent of men in the same survey see toes as sources of erotic pleasure.

The Chemical "O"

Sex involves the release of several hormones. These hormones enhance the sexual experience or intensify your feelings about your partner.

It should come as no surprise that orgasm triggers the release of mood-elevating hormones, known as endorphins, in the brain and spinal cord. The body's natural opiates, endorphins are the same chemicals that are released during vigorous exercise, contributing to a feeling of calm and well-being.

In recent years, researchers have focused attention on the role of a hormone called oxytocin. This chemical stimulates the smooth muscles and is responsible for the uterine contractions that occur with orgasm. Oxytocin also triggers orgasm by sensitizing the nerves to pleasurable sensations. Having an orgasm floods the body with even more oxytocin. At this stage of sexual response, the hormone's role is to reinforce the powerful feelings of affection and attachment you experience toward your partner, says Randy Thornhill, Ph.D., a biologist at the University of New Mexico in Albuquerque. The presence of oxytocin explains how having sex with someone intensifies our feelings for them. It also explains why we feel like cuddling after sex. It may even explain why many men succumb to the stereotypical post-sex stupor. (Women, it seems, produce more oxytocin in general and, thus, have a greater tolerance for its powerful effects.)

Oxytocin is a unique component of our evolutionary heritage, which appears to strengthen our social bonds. It is released by women during childbirth and breastfeeding. No wonder it's called the "cuddle chemical" or the "sociability hormone."

The Multiple "O"

Multiple orgasm means climaxing more than once during a single sexual act without having to completely stop and restart. Research conducted by Carol Darling, Ph.D., of the University of Florida at Tallahassee and J. Kenneth Davidson Sr., Ph.D., at the University of Wisconsin at Eau Claire indicates that nearly half of women are multiorgasmic, up from 14 percent when the Kinsey Institute asked women the same question in 1953. Darling and Davidson surveyed more than eight hundred women between the ages of twenty and sixty-five, from fifteen states. The multiorgasmic women they interviewed reported having from two to twenty orgasms within a single episode of foreplay, masturbation, or intercourse.

Sex researchers believe all women are capable of having multiple orgasms and that those who do may simply be more at ease with themselves sexually. If multiple orgasms have thus far eluded you and you want to explore the option, try this technique: Pause after climax and breathe rhythmically, continuing the stimulation. Keep in mind that multiple orgasms are not essential for satisfying, healthy sex.

The Blended "O"

Once you're familiar with your body's ability to orgasm, you can attempt the fancy stuff. Mix one vaginal orgasm with a clitoral orgasm and you've got what sex experts call a "blended" orgasm.

Some serious proponents of sexual pleasure seeking believe it's possible to extend the orgasmic response for an hour or more—in men and women. With the right technique—not to mention lots of spare time—you can launch a chain reaction in the muscles of the vagina, according to research by Alan Brauer, M.D., a psychiatrist in Palo Alto, California, and author of *Extended Sexual Orgasm* and *The ESO Ecstasy Program*. An extended, blended orgasm, Brauer says, is characterized by a long, continuous contraction punctuated by waves or phases—as opposed to the distinct and separate spasms that accompany multiple orgasms. "Instead of a squeezing there's a bearing down or a pushing out," he says. "Each of these push-out contractions are much longer." Brauer sees orgasmic response as a continuum—orgasmic women can teach themselves to be multiorgasmic, and multiorgasmic women can progress to blended orgasms with sufficient time, practice, and, most important, a willing partner.

The Evolutionary "O"

Orgasm has the obvious evolutionary purpose of keeping people interested in reproducing. But scientists have learned that subconscious evaluations of our sex partners probably plays a bigger role in sexual response than we ever knew.

Take the female orgasm. While male orgasm has an obvious reproductive function, scientists used to think that female orgasm was an accident of nature. Women can conceive without reaching orgasm, after all.

These views are changing, thanks to the pioneering work of British researchers, Robin Baker, Ph.D., and Mark Bellis, Ph.D., of the University of Manchester. Bellis and Baker found that female orgasm makes conception more likely. They asked volunteers to keep track of their orgasms and collect the fluid (called "flowback") that is expelled from the vagina after intercourse. They reported that when a woman climaxes anywhere from a minute before to forty-five minutes after her partner ejaculates, she retains much more sperm than she does when she has sex with no orgasm. The researchers concluded that women subconsciously control whether and when they climax to influence the probability of becoming pregnant. The ultimate goal: to secure the most favorable genes for their future offspring.

In other research, Randy Thornhill, the University of New Mexico biologist, and his colleague, psychologist Steve Gangestad, found that women make subconscious judgments of their male partners' symmetry—the extent to which the right and left sides of their bodies match up. (Symmetry, it seems, translates into better health and therefore superior genes.) Their studies show that women have more orgasms during sexual intercourse with men who are the most symmetrical. Amazingly, the degree of symmetrical differences we register subconsciously is undetectable to the naked eye.

The Faked "O"

The classic crowded deli scene from the movie *When Harry Met Sally* hilariously illustrates how easy it is to fake an earth-shattering orgasm. According to various surveys, up to 70 percent of women have played "the great pretender" at one time or another. Movies and television tell us that orgasm should be easy and fast. Not measuring up to these standards may make women feel inadequate—and more likely to fake.

"The majority of women have faked orgasms," says Marty Klein, Ph.D., a Palo Alto–based marriage counselor and sex therapist and author of the book *Ask Me Anything.* "It's understandable, considering the pressure men and women feel, and the ignorance both suffer with, about how to achieve orgasm."

Misrepresenting your sexual response is something you should think about carefully. "Ask yourself, When is it okay to lie to your mate? The same rules apply," Klein says.

That said, here are some other faking factors:

- *Pro:* Some women who have trouble reaching orgasm "act it out" until orgasm actually occurs. Pretending is a dress rehearsal for the real thing.
- *Con:* If you constantly fake orgasms, you never learn what really turns you on and how to experience the full pleasures of sex.
- *Pro:* Some therapists recognize that women sometimes fake orgasms to end sex gracefully. They're tired and don't want to hurt their partner's feelings. (Faking orgasm under these circumstances is potentially harmful, though, if pleasing your partner becomes more important than fulfilling your own needs for sexual satisfaction.)
- *Con:* Women who consistently fake orgasms may find it difficult to surrender to the real experience. Having an orgasm is among the most intimate things you can do with someone else. Faking can become a way around the intimacy.

The Elusive "O"

Studies have shown that about 10 percent of women do not have orgasms under any circumstances. Sex experts refer to this condition as anorgasmia.

Researchers roundly agree that many anorgasmic women are simply not getting enough stimulation and that most can be taught to climax. Women who have trouble reaching orgasm are often encouraged to take the time to explore what turns them on through masturbation. Masturbation allows a woman to discover what techniques may be pleasurable to her.

Anorgasmia may also signal an underlying health condition such as diabetes or a hormonal imbalance requiring medical attention. It might also be related to a traumatic sexual experience or a particularly repressive upbringing. A competent sex therapist can help in such cases.

THE "M" WORD: IN PRAISE OF MASTURBATION

Studies suggest that almost all men and women masturbate, but this harmless sex act is still taboo to some. The subject of masturbation is so loaded, it cost Jocelyn Elders, M.D., her job as U.S. Surgeon General when she straightforwardly suggested during the World AIDS Day Conference in 1994 that masturbation was a part of human sexuality.that might be taught.

It was another chapter in a rich, if troubled, history. The ancient Egyptians celebrated masturbation as the mode through which the Sun God, known as Atum, created the world's first couple, Shu and Tefnut. But by the time the Bible's Onan "spilt his seed" upon the ground, masturbation had become a sin against nature. The reputation has stuck. The Victorians may have considered masturbation to be a depraved and unnatural practice, but today we know that it—not to mention oral sex, homosexuality, and a score of other practices

---

once considered perverse—are common in the rest of the animal world, according to John Money, Ph.D., a sex researcher at Johns Hopkins University in Baltimore.

Today masturbation earns high marks as a sex therapy tool. It has proved one of the best ways to help women learn what is pleasurable to them and how to achieve orgasm. It is a simple sexual tension releaser—and the safest form of safe sex.

Studies show that people who masturbate are a sexually happier lot, on the whole. The "Sex in America" survey found that the frequency of masturbation does not decrease with marriage and that it is viewed by practitioners not as a substitute for but as an additional component of healthy sex. According to a 1991 study published in *The Journal of Sex Education and Therapy,* women who masturbate have significantly more orgasms, greater sexual desire, higher self-esteem, and greater marital satisfaction.

The No-Touch "O"

If women can climax spontaneously in their sleep, it follows that they might be able to induce orgasm through imagery alone. In her study of easily orgasmic women, Gina Ogden, Ph.D., author of *Women Who Love Sex,* reported that 64 percent of these women were able to climax the no-touch way, using imagery or fantasy. The physiological response was the same as women who climaxed through clitoral stimulation: Both sets of women experienced increases in blood pressure and heart rate, pupil dilation, and an enhanced tolerance for pain.

Obviously the no-touch orgasm is for women with vivid imaginations. But doing Kegel exercises during the fantasy session can help by triggering orgasmic contractions. Kegels (as they are simply called), named for the doctor who developed them, involve contracting and releasing the pubococcygeal (PC) muscle—the same one you would engage to stop the flow of urine. The PC runs from the front to the back of the pelvis. *(For a detailed Kegel regimen, see Chapter 6, page 149.)*

The Excedrin "O"

Orgasm is a great pain reliever, as many women have discovered when they masturbate to relieve the pain of menstrual cramps. Orgasm activates the release of a natural pain blocker. When a woman climaxes, her pain threshold can increase as much as 100 percent. Researchers have found that mere vaginal stimulation also blocks pain, and the pain-killing effect rises in proportion to the degree of stimulation.

Mo' Better Bliss

Learning what you like in bed and how your body responds to different stimuli are the bedrocks for a happy, satisfying sex life. Add a willing, giving partner and you're set to try these ideas for having more frequent and intense orgasms:

- *Develop a knowledge of your body.* Become aware of your body so you can communicate to your partner what you find pleasurable.
- *Build up steam* (if you build it, you will come). Practice start-stop sexual stimulation: Have your partner focus on your clitoris for awhile, then switch to your vaginal hot spots. Then return again to the clitoris. Hovering on the brink of orgasm for a time can make your eventual climax even more powerful and satisfying.
- *Position yourself.* Be willing to change places and try different positions. The rear vaginal entry and female-on-top positions are

thought to be particularly useful for triggering vaginal and multiple orgasms.

- *Exercise your love muscle.* Studies show that strengthening the PC muscle intensifies orgasm. You can do this by practicing Kegel exercises *(see Chapter 8, page 149).*

Taking Matters into Your Own Hands

Betty Dodson's classic self-help primer, *Sex for One: The Joy of Self-Loving,* is an explicit and informative lesson in masturbation. Her videos, *Self-Loving* and *Celebrating Orgasm,* feature techniques for enhancing orgasms through masturbation. Write to Betty Dodson, P.O. Box 1933, Murray Hill Station, New York, NY 10156. *First Person Sexual,* a series of essays on self-pleasuring, edited by Joani Blank (Down There Press, 1996, $14.50), reconsiders societal attitudes toward solo sex.

The New Intercourse

Fewer than half of women have orgasms during sexual intercourse, but a sex therapist has developed a way to improve that statistic—a sexual technique called coital alignment technique, or C.A.T. After New York sex researcher Edward Eichel taught his technique to couples, the percentage of women clients who achieved orgasm regularly through intercourse rose from about 25 percent to more than 75 percent. Other researchers have confirmed his results.

The C.A.T. differs from traditional intercourse by providing stimulation to the clitoris and G-spot simultaneously. With all of this going for the C.A.T., it's not surprising that the frequency of simultaneous orgasm soars from 5 to 50 percent after couples master the technique. Here's how it works:

Start in the traditional male-on-top position, but have your partner rest his weight on you, instead of his elbows. He then shifts his body forward about two inches so that his pelvis is placed over yours. The base of the penis presses against your clitoris. Instead of thrusting, you move your hips together rhythmically using a rocking motion.

Unlike traditional thrusting, in which the clitoris receives no or only intermittent contact, the C.A.T. is intended to provide continuous clitoral stimulation. But it may require patience and practice. "The position doesn't work without coordinated movement," Eichel says. "While the man and woman alternately lead the upper and downward stroke of sexual movement, they maintain clitoral contact exerting continuous pressure and counterpressure genitally." (The C.A.T. should not be confused with a position called "riding high," which refers to a specific position without the clitoral choreography.)

Turn-ons and Titillations

Sexual tastes and tolerances are as varied as our appetites for foods. At one end of the sexual spectrum are bizarre sexual fetishes—from acrotomophilia (an unusual attraction to amputees) to zoophilia (sex with animals). The *Encyclopedia of Sex* lists 102 such so-called paraphilias. At the other end are commonplace sex acts such as masturbation, oral sex, sexual fantasizing, or anal sex.

"We can talk about something being unusual, but the truth is that most of what our culture considers deviant is not that unusual," says Marty Klein, Ph.D.

Social mores influence both your attitude toward sex and the types of behaviors you consider acceptable. Whether you feel comfortable with your sexual desires also depends to a great extent on your individual moral code. Many sex therapists believe that a sexual practice is aberrant only if it interferes with the rest of your life or is harmful to yourself or others.

A healthy love life can incorporate many stimuli—from tattoos to G-strings, phone sex to computer sex, videos to vibrators. And a growing body of research shows that women are as diverse in their sexual desires as men. This section explores the latest research and trends in sexual expression.

When Fancy Turns to Fantasy

Steamy kisses on a beach at sunset . . . Seduction by a long-lost lover . . . Torrid sex in an elevator with a stranger—make that two strangers . . .

Welcome to the world of sex fantasies. Like dreams, fantasies are windows to the soul. Sexual fantasies reveal our most personal sexual yearnings—yearnings that may be too private for public consumption, fantasies sometimes too private even for our partners. Which may explain the persistence of certain myths about fantasy, such as women don't fantasize about sex, for instance, or fantasizing signals an inadequate sex life.

Research indicates that most of us—some 95 percent of men and women—fantasize. People who fantasize frequently have more sex with a greater number of sexual partners and engage in a greater variety of erotic experiences. Not only is fantasizing about sex compatible with a healthy sex life, experts say, but failing to fantasize is actually associated with sexual problems.

The most common fantasies for men and women:

- Having sex with a past, current, or imaginary lover, especially a stranger or other "forbidden" partner.
- Being completely irresistible to someone.
- Engaging in exotic sexual practices or positions.
- Overpowering someone—or being overpowered.

Contrary to common wisdom, women like to think about sex almost as often as men. But the latest research shows that women's fantasies have a fundamentally different focus, says Harold Leitenberg, Ph.D., a professor of psychology at the University of Vermont at Burlington, who reviewed more than two hundred studies on sexual fantasy and published his analysis in a 1995 issue of *Psychological Bulletin*. He found that women's fantasies more often focused on the sensual side of sex, took place in romantic settings, and emphasized the emotional aspects of sex. They also unfolded at a slower pace. Men's fantasies contained more explicit and visual images, more anonymous sex, and more sexual partners.

Women focus on emotional characteristics of imagined partners; men focus on physical characteristics. Women describe romantic, passionate interludes; men focus on numerous sex acts. Women imagine things being done to them; men imagine doing them. "Men tend to play a more active or dominant role than women in many of the fantasies," Leitenberg says. "They are also more likely to have multiple partners and conjure up specific physical attributes than women. Women, on the other hand, tend to stick to fairly romantic story lines." Small wonder that men turn to *Penthouse* and women to Harlequin romances when seeking vicarious sexual thrills.

Both women and men have domination and submission fantasies. But whereas women fantasize about being overpowered by an amorous lover, men tend to imagine overpowering a willing, lustful female. Forty-four percent of men have fantasized about dominating a partner, while 51 percent of women fantasize about being forced to have sex.

This does not suggest, Leitenberg cautions, that women want to be raped in real life. In their daydreams, women have control over what happens, and their fantasies do not typically involve violence or brutality. "Many women have these sorts of fantasies, but it doesn't mean she has any sort of psychological problem. Rape fantasies are mainly about the man being so overwhelmed with desire because the woman is attractive that he can't help himself. And the woman desires it, too," Leitenberg says. "It's akin to the 'swept-off-her-feet' passion of romantic novels."

About a quarter of fantasizers feel guilty about their fantasies. But sex therapists would like to relieve them of this burden: Many say fantasies can actually improve sexual relationships. Imagining that you are doing something is a far cry from actually doing it. Many experts actually prescribe it as a way to enhance sensual awareness during sex with your regular partner. And the data suggest that fantasizers who succumb to guilt have less sex—and less pleasure.

"Sexual fantasy is not a form of cheating. The mind is just part of the complicated arousal system of sex," Leitenberg says. "It is healthy. It does you no harm."

What else does the research say?

- Fantasizing usually begins between the ages of 11 and 13. Sexual fantasies are more common in youth, growing less frequent with age.
- The sexual fantasies of gay men and lesbians have the same content as heterosexuals, only they see themselves with partners of the same sex.
- Although men and women fantasize in equal numbers, men have more frequent fantasies than women.

Women and Erotica

Fantasy isn't the only arena of sexuality that is getting an attitude overhaul. Women are also coming out of the closet about their interest in erotic literature and films. In fact, women rent more than a quarter of adult entertainment videos each year.

Not everyone is comfortable with the trend. "Our culture is not comfortable with female sexuality in general," explains Marty Klein, Ph.D. "And pornography basically shows women as wanting sex, enjoying sex, asking for it, and experiencing pleasure."

Many of us grew up thinking that pornographic material was bad for women. Pornographic films, magazines, and books have often portrayed women in a questionable light—on the receiving end of male force and aggression.

One of the fastest growing trends in porn promises to be more palatable: erotic books and movies created for women from a woman's perspective. "I've been working for ten years in this field and there's a noticeable boom in women-written and -published erotica in which the emphasis is on female orgasm and pleasure. There's a broad range of material about women from diverse backgrounds and ages," says Cathy Winks, a salesperson at Good Vibrations, a sex toy and video emporium in San Francisco, and coauthor of the *Good Vibrations Guide to Sex*.

Women are feeling freer to express their own interest in erotica. "This is an idea that's evolving," Winks says. "Opposition to pornography is not a knee-jerk response for many young women, largely because there's an increasing amount that is for and by women."

What exactly constitutes erotica, anyway—and what is pornographic? This question comes down to individual tastes. "Everyone has their own distinctions: If it turns me on, it's erotica. If it turns me off, it's porn," Winks quips. The point is that there's nothing wrong with enjoying erotic materials, and women who are turned on by them need not worry that doing so is politically—or sexually—incorrect.

The New Erotica

What can you expect if you sample the new erotic material for women? Like female fantasies, some of these films and books emphasize the emotional and romantic sides to sex and give equal time to foreplay and nongenital touch. Many give voice to the full range and fulfillment of women's natural sexual desires and responses.

Many sex therapists believe that women-centered erotica affirms female sexuality. It allows women to acknowledge their sexual needs, and it even provides a way to satisfy them. Indeed, sexually explicit films can provide a blueprint for future intimate encounters, expanding your sexual repertoire with ideas and techniques you never thought of.

For some, pornography fills the gap created by our culture's scanty approach to sex education because it demonstrates diverse sexual styles and positions. It can also provide the fodder for future fantasies that add spice to sex. In other words, porn has a place in a healthy sex life.

It's how you use it that really matters. If sexually explicit materials are the only way you can express your sexuality, there could be a problem.

Under these circumstances porn can reduce intimacy. Porn can also undermine a woman's sexual self-confidence if she compares herself with the image on the screen and finds herself lacking. Some female-centered films, however, feature women of all shapes, sizes, and races. Like any genre, the new erotica is of wildly varying levels of quality and taste. Major book publishers now regularly publish erotica, as well. Look for works edited by Susie Bright and Joani Blank. Women-friendly erotic film companies include K.P.C. Productions, Deborah Films, and Femme Productions.

Sex Sales

With its pink-and-white walls and colorful art, you might mistake Eve's Garden for a bath shop or an upscale gift boutique. A closer examination of the store's shelves reveals more unusual wares: edible body paints, massage oils, and pink vibrators. These items leave the store discreetly hidden in feminine flowered bags.

Female-oriented sex businesses like Eve's Garden suggest that sex toys have left the sleazy sexual fringe and established a firm foothold in the mainstream. In fact, more women are finding that sex props are another way to expand their sexual horizons.

The first of its kind, Eve's Garden—located a few blocks from Manhattan's Times Square—is now only one of a dozen or so women-centered sex stores. Dell Williams started the store in 1974, on the heels of the women's movement, to provide a safe haven for women to explore new paths to pleasure. Her goal: to give women the okay and the opportunity to discover their sexuality.

Other women-run sex shops have followed suit, including Good Vibrations of San Francisco, which runs a thriving mail-order business. *(See "Mail Order Sources for Sexual Toys and Erotica," page 119.)*

Here are some of the more popular types of sexual wares:

Vibrators

Vibrators are shedding their low-rent reputation these days, and for a good reason. Vibrators are a sure way to reach orgasm and are responsible for many a woman's first climax. Things to remember if you're in the market: Vibrators come either with an electric cord or are battery-powered. The trade-off is that the corded vibrators offer more power but are limited by their cord length. For years electric massagers have been marketed for use in relaxing tense muscles. Other vibrators are clearly intended for sexual play. For example, some handheld units look like phalluses and are designed for insertion. Vibrator varieties include multispeed and wearable units, such as a vibrating penis ring that sends pleasure waves to both parties, and even a remote-controlled vibrator. The "Cadillac" of corded models is the Hitachi Magic Wand, a twenty-year best-seller that's used by sex therapists.

Everything you ever wanted to know about vibrators—from types to techniques—can be found in the informative videotape *Good Vibrations: An Explicit Guide to Vibrators* ($32.50). Write: Blank Tapes, P.O. Box 8263, Emeryville, CA 94608; 510-655-7399, 510-655-3351 (fax).

Edibles

Though most of these products would not fly with a gourmet, edible sex products can add new dimensions to sex. Chocolate body paint and honey-flavored body powders and creams are among the best of the edibles. Other products feature flavors like piña colada, strawberry, cherry, peach, or cinnamon. Or simply try real foods such as Jell-O, honey, chocolate, or whipped cream.

Massage Oils

Any scented oil can turn massage into an erotic experience by enhancing the sensuousness of lovemaking. Choose from floral scents, such as lavender or rose, or botanical aromas like rosemary, sandalwood, or herbal blends. Essential oils, which are concentrated and, therefore, more intense, should be diluted first as they can be harmful to the skin in their pure form. Always test the oil first on a small patch of skin for possible reactions.

New Condom Choices

Look for festive, jewel-toned condoms in colors like purple and pink or condoms coated with flavored lubricants. Sheik brand mint-flavored condoms, coated with a dry mint powder that tastes like spearmint gum, have been unofficially voted the best-tasting condom for four years running by employees of Condomania (800-9–CONDOM), a chain of condom stores. If you or your partner has an allergy to latex, try Avanti, a new condom made of polyurethane, or Reality, the polyurethane condom designed for women.

Sex Wear

Sex props run the gamut from fake-fur-lined blindfolds and outrageous feather-trimmed mules to hard-core items like nipple clamps and studded collars. Costumes can help you play out your favorite fantasy.

Individual tastes run from the romantic (Victoria's Secret–style satin or silk negligees and camisoles) to the risqué (G-strings, leather harnesses, whips and chains). Some women enjoy using feathers as a part of fore-play or lovemaking; others like brandishing whips. Anything goes, depending on your inclinations and comfort level.

Sex Props: Basic Health and Hygiene

Silicone Toys: In between uses, toys made of silicone, such as dildos, should be cleaned with warm water and an unscented detergent. To sterilize, submerge in boiling water for no longer than five to eight minutes. This is especially important if the item has been used anally. You can also place silicone products in the top rack of the dishwasher. Dry the items thoroughly before putting them away to deter bacterial growth. To avoid infections, it's a wise idea to roll a condom over the toy, especially if you are going to share it with a partner.

Vinyl Toys: Clean with a warm cloth and mild soap. Use a condom with the toy if you want to be especially careful.

Vibrators: Good Vibrations recommends wiping them clean with a cloth moistened with warm water or alcohol. Vinyl parts can be cleaned in the top dishwasher rack provided they have no mechanical or electrical hardware. Never immerse the vibrator in water; the motor's parts can corrode. Condoms will keep vibrators cleaner—and healthier. Wand-style vibrators are not meant for penetration. Only use models specially designed for anal use in the rectum, since there is a chance you may be unable to retrieve small vibrators.

Rubber Dildos and Wands: Since rubber is porous, your best bet is to roll a condom over these props before using. Use mild soap and water and dry thoroughly before storing.

Harnesses, G-Strings, and Other Intimate Apparel: Wash items as you would any delicate garment. Dry before storing.

Mindful Sex

The hottest trend in sexual bliss, tantric sex, is thousands of years old. More people are turning to ancient tantric and other Eastern sexual traditions to improve the quality of their lovemaking and deepen the bonds of intimacy with their partners.

"Asian techniques can increase sexual enhancement, so both partners have a more deeply fulfilling experience on many different levels—sensual, emotional, and spiritual," says Harrison Voight, Ph.D., of the California Institute of Integral Studies in San Francisco. Historically, tantra combined sexuality and meditation as a means to spiritual enlightenment. Whether or not enlightenment is your goal, tantric principles promise to shift the focus of sex away from performance and toward connection.

Tantric sex may require holding back orgasm, a principle that seems woefully at odds with our orgasm-obsessed Western sexuality. But proponents believe tantric sex heightens orgasmic response while strengthening your relationship. "The techniques help transform the typical Western approach to sex, which is orgasm oriented, into a fuller, deeper, and more meaningful experience," says Voight, who offers five simple tantric "explorations" for enhancing sex.

- **Create a ritual.** Devise a unique and personal prelude to sex. A formal transition to intimate behavior helps you shift gears. Try bathing, feeding, or massaging each other, and lighting special candles. Focus on the details of your surroundings, including the lights and sounds.
- **Synchronize your breathing.** Concentrating on your own and your partner's breath is a sure method for shutting out distracting thoughts and preoccupations and intensifying the connection between you and your partner.
- **Sustain eye contact.** This technique is surprisingly powerful. "Fixing one's gaze into a partner's eyes throughout all phases of the sexual exchange can lead to a merging of oceanic dimension," Voight says. You may feel awkward at first, since this practice runs counter to the Western way of closing our eyes during sex. But the practice becomes easier—and more rewarding—with practice.
- **Have motionless intercourse.** Heterosexual couples can experiment with stopping the motion shortly after the penis enters the vagina. Homosexual couples can bring a halt to the action at some other peak point of sexual contact. For example, the activity that becomes the so-called still point can be a deep kiss or the cupping of a breast. In either case, the stillness provides a striking contrast

to the motion typically associated with lovemaking. The quiet time can vary from a minute at first to longer periods over time.

- **Have sex without orgasm.** The hallmark of tantric sex, this principle involves refraining from orgasm to cultivate the sensual experience of sex. The tantric exercise entails exploring all the dimensions of sexual contact that are possible without orgasm. Removing orgasm from sex may sound frustrating, but it can open you to a new experience of sex and a new sense of closeness with your partner.

Yummy Sex?

Sometimes you need a little novelty to bypass sexual boredom. The next time you're feeling ho-hum about sex, try the Yab-Yum, a sexy Tibetan posture. Using the technique, a man and woman sit facing each other, she on his lap, her legs crossed behind his back, his legs folded under her. Gaze into each other's eyes, coordinate your breathing, and let sexuality soar.

The New Aphrodisiacs

What do ginseng, garlic, oysters, ground rhinoceros tusks, and chocolate have in common? They are just a few of the items humans have used to boost libido and sexual pleasure.

Named for the Greek goddess Aphrodite, who personified physical love, aphrodisiacs are as old as civilization. Over the centuries humans have made a habit of imbuing natural substances with lust-restoring properties, especially those that resembled sexual organs. This explains both the enduring mystique of oysters and the disappearance of the rhinoceros, whose coveted tusks are ground into a fine dust and used by many people in the Far East to heighten sexual performance.

Aphrodisiacs are categorized as having either a biochemical or psychological effect. Under this broad definition, pornography and fantasy clearly are aphrodisiacs. For that matter, anything that one believes sparks sexual interest probably does.

This is one reason that there is virtually no scientific evidence to substantiate the love-promoting properties of common aphrodisiacs, including many herbs now aggressively advertised for these effects. Proving that sex remedies are effective is more difficult than it seems. Since the brain is the primary organ involved in sexual arousal, sex researchers have to rule out the placebo effect of a study—the process by which stimulation might occur from simply believing that a particular sex cure is effective.

In some cases advertised aphrodisiacs are not merely ineffective, but are known to be dangerous. For instance, cantharis, also known as Spanish fly, involves some serious health risks when used in excess. Made of dried beetles, Spanish fly stimulates the genitals by irritating the urinary tract. It is capable of causing burns and infections. An over-the-counter topical aphrodisiac, identified as a Chinese herb called Chan Su, caused the deaths of four New York men between 1993 and 1995. The substance contains naturally occurring steroids, which apparently triggered heart arrhythmias in the men. The FDA has issued rulings stating that no over-the-counter aphrodisiac drug product is recognized as safe and effective.

Research has focused on several substances and strategies that may prove to be effective, however, and many people swear by other sex-enhancing products that appear to cause no harm. Here's a look at the current and future offerings:

Pharmaceutical Love Potions

Promising sexual aids could come from the labs of pharmacologists working on drugs that act on the brain's "sex center" in the hypothalamus. Research has revealed that drugs that interact with receptors for dopamine, a chemical messenger in the brain, appear to stimulate sex drive. In fact, low sexual desire has been linked to low levels of dopamine. Drugs that reverse this deficiency include two medications that treat Parkinson's disease, Eldepryl and L-Dopa, and the antidepressant Wellbutrin. Other antidepressants, such as Prozac, Zoloft, and Paxil, often have the opposite effect of depressing sexual interest. *(See "Prescriptions for Problems," page 138.)*

Researchers are tentatively exploring the use of oxytocin, the so-called cuddle chemical, which plays a crucial role in sexual response. But so far they have been stymied by the problem of finding a method of delivering the drug effectively. Their efforts are aimed primarily at restoring sexual function in those who have lost it due to medical or psychological problems, rather than those with normal sexuality who seek an extra boost in bed.

Foods

If popular aphrodisiacs like oysters and chocolate enhance ardor, they probably do so because you expect them to. Most experts don't place much stock in the sex-boosting power of foods, favoring old-fashioned good nutrition instead. (So much for an instant sexual boost.) Eating a low-fat diet will help keep your arteries and blood flow in good working condition, which translates into robust sexual response. Abundant intake of antioxidants, the nutrition superstars found in fresh vegetables and fruits, should prevent your sexual anatomy from prematurely aging—along with the rest of your body. Some Japanese researchers have reported that spirulina, a blue-green alga, activates the production of sexual hormones, but their work has yet to be replicated in American labs.

Herbs

Yohimbine, a popular herb made from the bark of an African tree, is widely prescribed by physicians for impotence. It seems to stimulate the nerve centers in the brain that control erections. Some studies have shown effectiveness in men with erectile dysfunction but no libido-boosting effects in a control group. Researchers have become increasingly wary of its potentially dangerous side effects because it plays havoc with some patients' blood pressure. Other intriguing herbs include saw palmetto and damiana, a shrub found in Mexico. Kava-kava, guarana, licorice, ginseng, golden seal, nux vomica, and gotu kola also fall into the probably harmless, potentially helpful, category of herbal products available for use as aphrodisiacs.

The Sex-Exercise Connection

There is no lack of evidence for the idea that exercise acts as an aphrodisiac. Common sense says that when you're feeling fit and attractive, intimacy is more appealing. According to several large studies involving men and women, the results of regular workouts are undeniably sexy: more frequent sex, an increase in orgasms, and greater sexual pleasure in general. Consider these research hightlights:

- A study at Chicago State University of five hundred women found that 58 percent reported greater contentment with their "sexual selves" because of exercise. Twenty-five percent said they experienced arousal or orgasm while working out, and 30 percent reported a leap in libido immediately following exercise.
- In a recent runner's poll, 83 percent of the female respondents and 75 percent of males claimed that running enhanced their sex life.

Seventy-nine percent of the women and 72 percent of the men reported that running makes them more sexually responsive.

- A survey of eight thousand women by Los Angeles psychologist Linda De Villers, Ph.D., showed that 31 percent found exercise led to more frequent sexual activity, and 40 percent said their ability to become aroused had increased since they began an exercise program. More than 25 percent of the respondents reported an enhanced ability to achieve orgasm, while a few even reported that their orgasms were more intense.
- A study at the University of California at San Diego revealed that middle-aged men made love more frequently and had more satisfying sex as well as an increase in orgasms after nine months on a vigorous exercise program.

Experts point to a host of physiological changes that may explain the "sexual second wind" that comes with physical exertion. Exercise triggers levels of mood-elevating endorphins and elevates production of testosterone, the hormone most closely associated with sexual function in both men and women. These short-term chemical changes could explain the postworkout libido benefit. Moreover, many fitness activities, such as swimming and dancing, are eros enhancing—that is, they have a sensuous aspect that contributes to greater body awareness and sexual arousal.

Over time, physical fitness helps all your body's systems function better—sexual systems included. Exercise confers important cardiovascular benefits, improving the circulation of blood into the pelvic region and genitals. Regular aerobic exercise helped men at the University of California at San Diego lower the ratio of "bad" LDL to "good" HDL cholesterol, improving their capacity for climax. Weight training strengthens the muscles that support the body during sex and improves agility, allowing for greater ease of movement.

The physical benefits of exercise often lead to an erotic attitude adjustment. According to DeVillers, women and men who exercise nearly always claim greater self-, and sexual, confidence with regular workouts. Self-image often undergoes a positive shift, and fitness seekers develop a healthy sense of respect for their bodies, which has a ripple effect on sexuality. "These are people who feel good about the way they look physically. That can have a pretty positive effect on sexuality," says Phillip Whitten, Ph.D., a Harvard University anthropologist and author of a study of sexuality in a group of older swimmers.

Exercise has been shown to alleviate depression and feelings of worthlessness, which inevitably boosts sexual pleasure. "In general, depressed people aren't very interested in sex," says Marjorie Schulte, director of the Schulte Institute for Psychotherapy and Human Sexuality in Scottsdale, Arizona. "Exercising and feeling good about yourself stimulate sexual desire."

Achieving Sexual Fitness

Cardiovascular conditioning, the cornerstone of any good exercise program, is the only thing that can equip you with the endurance needed for healthy lovemaking. Swimming, running, biking, aerobics classes, and brisk walking are favorite forms of aerobic exercise, which gets your heart rate up—along with your sexual appetite. Be sure to cool down after intense exertion to prevent muscle strain and dizziness.

A program of moderate weight training can help build stamina for sex and strengthen and tone the arms, legs, chest, and back. The focus should be on increasing repetitions rather than lifting greater weight. Try crunches to strengthen the abdomen and back. Inner thigh stretches will keep you limber in the right places. Like good nutrition, exercise must become a habit to be of use as an intimacy enhancer. (If you have been sedentary, consult with a health-care professional before starting any exercise program.)

Resources

Books and Other Publications

A New View of a Woman's Body (Feminist Health Press, 8240 Santa Monica Boulevard, Los Angeles, CA 90046; 213-650-1508).

The G-Spot and Other Recent Discoveries About Human Sexuality, by A. K. Ladas, B. Whipple, and J. D. Perry (New York: Dell 1983).

The Art of Sexual Ecstasy: The Path of Sacred Sexuality for Western Lovers, by Margo Anand (Jeremy P. Tarcher, 1989).

Anne Hooper's Ultimate Sex Guide CD-ROM: A Sex Therapist's Personalized Program for Enriching Your Sex Life (Dorling Kindersley Multimedia, 1996).

The Good Vibrations Guide to Sex, by Cathy Winks and Anne Semans (Cleis Press, 1994).

Anal Pleasure and Health, by Jack Morin, Ph.D. (Down There Press, 1998).

Sex-Related Research

The Kinsey Institute for Research in Sex, Gender and Reproduction
Indiana University
Morrison House 313
Bloomington, IN 47405-2501
812-855-7686

Mail Order Sources for Sexual Toys and Erotica

Good Vibrations
Sexuality Library Book and Videostore
938 Howard Street, Suite 101
San Francisco, CA 94103
800-289-8423, 415-974-8990
Videos, sex toys, and books by mail, or visit the store.

Eve's Garden
119 W. Fifty-seventh Street, Suite 420
New York, NY 10019
800-848-3837, 212-757-8651
A discreet place for women to buy sex videos and props.

Blowfish
2261 Market Street, #284
San Francisco, CA 94114
415-285-6064
Mail-order erotica with a feminine focus.

Grand Opening
318 Harvard Street, Suite 32
Arcade Building, Coolidge Corner
Brookline, MA 02146
617-731-2626
Web site: /http://www.grandopening.com
A woman-oriented sexuality boutique.

Toys in Babeland
711 East Pike Street
Seattle, WA 98122
800-658-9119, 206-328-2914
Web site: /http://www.babeland.com
A sex toy shop run by women for women.

Trashy Lingerie
402 North La Cienega Boulevard
Los Angeles, CA 90048
310-652-4543
Sex "warehouse" with extensive selection of costumes, lingerie, and props.

Womyn's Ware Inc.
896 Commercial Drive
Vancouver, BC V5L 3Y5, Canada
604-254-2543
Web site: /http://www.womynsware.com
Offers sex products that celebrate women's sexuality.

Passion Flower
4 Yosemite Avenue
Oakland, CA 94611
510-601-7750
A woman-focused erotic supply store.

It's My Pleasure
3106 North East Sixty-fourth Boulevard
Portland, OR 97213
503-280-8080
Sex toys, books, cards, and music with a female theme.

6 | Sexual Saboteurs

What do infection, negative emotions, illness, douching, stress, medications, fatigue, and spermicide have in common? Each of these factors can interfere with healthy, loving sex. Considering all the possible pitfalls, it's a wonder anyone gets as far as foreplay.

Sex is such a taboo topic that when problems occur, women often keep the details to themselves. In a recent study, only 3 percent of patients volunteered that they were having difficulties with sex. But when directly asked about sexual woes, nearly one in five confessed to a problem, according to Anita Nelson, M.D., associate professor in obstetrics and gynecology at Harbor–UCLA Medical Center in Los Angeles.

Most sex stoppers have solutions, however, and no woman need tolerate poor sexual functioning. "The quality of life is greatly affected for better or worse by sexual expression and control," says Domeena C. Renshaw, M.D., director of the Loyola Sexual Dysfunction Clinic in Maywood, Illinois.

The first step toward keeping your sex life lively is to learn how your body works and identify the conditions under which it works best. Then you will know how to keep it in good working order. You can also be alert to such intimacy enemies as vaginal infections, urinary tract problems, and sexually acquired diseases.

The good news is that there is more information available to help you accomplish these tasks. After years of neglect, women's health and sexuality are finally getting some long overdue attention from medical researchers. The data are shaking up many long-held beliefs about the causes and treatments of sex-stalling diseases and conditions while identifying some unexpected sex stoppers. This sexual health information is slowly trickling down to doctors who treat patients. In the meantime, you can take advantage of these research gains and help yourself to greater sexual health.

Good Bugs, Bad Bugs

The first concept you need to understand to stay sexually fit—and happy in bed—is the idea of a vaginal "ecology." Gynecological researchers, spurred by new data, have been pushing this way of thinking about the vagina. Not simply a place for penises, babies, and tampons, the vagina is also home to a variety of microscopic organisms that conspire to make it the cleanest spot in the body, according to Sharon Hillier, M.D., director of Reproductive Infectious Disease Research at Magee–Women's Hospital at the University of Pittsburgh.

Like a tropical rain forest, the vagina is a complex and self-regulating "ecosystem." The primary players in this ecological complex are friendly bacteria called lactobacilli. When the system is running properly, these canny creatures constantly manufacture hydrogen peroxide, in effect churning out small amounts of bleach to keep less than desirable organisms—like the bacteria responsible for infections and STDs—in check.

The idea of a naturally clean vagina is so at odds with society's and women's own beliefs that Hillier has been taking to the road on a virtual vagina campaign. "The healthy vaginal ecosystem," she declares to physician groups, magazine reporters, and FDA panels, "is an endangered habitat."

Yeast and unhealthy bacteria can disturb the natural balance if given the opportunity to grow. Modern American women provide plenty of opportunities—by inappropriately treating themselves with nonprescription yeast cures, douching, or having multiple sexual partners who help introduce harmful new bugs into the previously pristine environment by wiping out the good lactobacilli. Simply taking a course of antibiotics can trigger a yeast overgrowth. Each of these scenarios sets the stage for potential problems.

Ironically, one of the primary culprits in many "eco-gynecological" disasters are products aimed at helping women feel "fresh" and "sexy." Douches, vaginal deodorants, even scented panty liners, contain chemicals that can irritate the vaginal walls, disrupt the normal flora, and allow bad bugs to flourish—which can lead to very unsexy infections.

According to a 1996 study of women conducted at the University of Washington in Seattle, for example, women who routinely douched for hygiene were four times more likely to lose their healthful lactobacilli in the year and a half following the study. "Women who douche thinking it will clean them can upset their ecosystem in much the same way as putting weed killer on the lawn can kill the underlying lawn," Hillier says. "It has no medical benefits." Douching, in fact, is associated with an increased risk for pelvic inflammatory disease (PID). (Evidence also suggests that talc-based powders and deodorant sprays may increase the risk for ovarian cancer.)

Researchers suspect that women past menopause may face new risks for ecosystem imbalances as the vagina becomes drier, less elastic, and more prone to trauma in the absence of estrogen. Though data on rates of infection in these women is slim, Hillier says that "most doctors would agree that estrogen replacement will keep the vagina in a healthier state."

The good news for women of all ages is that the vagina has a natural tendency to restore itself—to a point: Gynecologists warn that odor—particularly a fishy odor—is almost always a tip-off to the presence of an infection requiring medical attention.

Anything that harms vaginal health can undermine intimacy by making intercourse uncomfortable or even painful. What could be worse for your sex life? The wise course is to become familiar with the common sexual saboteurs before they strike.

Vaginal Irritation

Vaginal irritation may foster infection, but it can also be a symptom, so it makes sense to identify its source. Vaginal products, including douches and chemical contraceptives—indeed, almost anything that can be put in or near the vagina—may bother some women, causing redness or itching, and derailing sex. If this happens, stop using the product, let nature take its course, and take comfort in the fact that a true allergic reaction is rare.

Fortunately, tampons seem to have little effect on the vaginal ecology. In a study published in the *Journal of Infectious Diseases,* researchers found that tampons did not adversely affect the vaginal ecosystem, and tampon users were at no greater risk for infections than nonusers. In fact, today's tampons are far safer than in the past. The super absorbent, synthetic tampons that spurred an epidemic of toxic shock syndrome in the early 1980s are no longer on the market. (These tampons irritated the vaginal walls, promoting the growth of a lethal form of Staphylococcus bacteria.)(See Chapter 3, *"Tampons and Toxic Shock Syndrome,"* page 47.)

Irritation can also affect the external genital area, the vulva. This is a typical site for dermatitis, a skin condition that causes dryness and itching and is often due to tight or chafing clothes. "It's a result of the retention of heat combined with the moisture of normal vaginal secretions," says Peter Lynch, M.D., chairman of the Department of Dermatology at the University of California at Davis, a specialist in vulvar dermatology. The solution: Keep the area cooler and drier by wearing loose-fitting clothes. Your doctor may prescribe a steroid ointment if the area becomes inflamed.

Infections: The Usual Suspects

Add discharge and odor to your complaint list and you're probably looking at a vaginal infection, commonly termed vaginitis. The sources of infection—bacteria, yeast, or a wily parasite—may be microscopic, but they have a mighty way of sabotaging your sexual pleasure.

The problem is, some women don't recognize the symptoms, blame themselves for bad hygiene, and try to hide unpleasant smells with scented products that aggravate the infection. "Normal secretions are not foul or fishy," says David E. Soper, M.D., director of the Division of Benign Gynecology at the Medical University of South Carolina.

Doctors are often party to the cover-up. In a recent Gallup survey, nearly 50 percent of the physicians surveyed reported that they did not treat the most common infection, bacterial vaginosis (BV) if patients didn't complain of symptoms—even when the doctors found evidence of infection.

It's a mistake to assume that vaginitis will be caught as a matter of course during a routine gynecological visit. "Many women think the purpose of the Pap smear is to identify infections," says Jill Maura Rabin, M.D., assistant professor of obstetrics and gynecology at Albert Einstein College of Medicine in New York. On the contrary, the Pap smear was designed to pick up cervical cell changes and is not a good screening tool for vaginal infections. Therefore, it's important to speak up about troublesome symptoms such as odors and discharge.

Gynecological researchers have waged a campaign among doctors to have routine screening for vaginitis included in the annual pelvic exam. If your doctor does not, and you believe you may be at risk for vaginal infections, ask to be tested. "These tests are simple, easy to do, and take pennies to perform," says Edward Hook III, professor of medicine at the University of Alabama at Birmingham.

The consequences of unchecked vaginal infections now appear to be more dangerous than doctors previously believed and can contribute to pelvic inflammatory disease (PID) and pregnancy complications. "There is a transition from seeing vaginal problems as a nuisance to seeing them as a menace," Hillier says.

These vaginal infections are the most common:

Bacterial Vaginosis (BV)

BV often produces an increase in discharge that is thin, grayish or white, and has a foul, fishy odor, especially after intercourse. (Normal vaginal secretions are white and clear.) It is sometimes accompanied by itching and irritation.

BV is responsible for 12 million office visits each year and affects some 15 percent of all women. (In women who douche, the percentage may be as high as 30 percent; among monogamous women who don't douche it is probably around 5 percent.) Triggered by an overgrowth of normally occurring bacteria in the vagina, it's due to any one of a number of factors known to disrupt the vaginal ecosystem, including douching, sexual intercourse, sometimes even barrier contraceptives such as diaphragms.

BV has recently been linked to a higher rate of pelvic inflammatory disease (PID), postoperative infections, and abnormal cell growth. According to James McGregor, M.D., vice chairman and professor of obstetrics and gynecology at the University of Colorado Health Science Center, BV is also associated with preterm birth and premature rupture of the membranes, leakage of amniotic fluid before labor has begun. In a National Institutes of Health study of more than thirteen thousand pregnant women, those with BV in the twenty-third to twenty-eighth week of pregnancy were 40 percent more likely to deliver a low-birth-weight baby (under five pounds). BV is also believed to facilitate the movement of STDs, such as gonorrhea and chlamydia, into the fallopian tubes.

For these reasons, getting diagnosed and treated is critical. The prescription drugs metronidazole (administered orally or vaginally) or clindamycin will usually do the trick. (Avoid drinking alcohol until twenty-four hours after you finish the drug regimen.)

Many women reach for a nonprescription yeast treatment at any sign of discharge. But doctors warn that they do not work for BV and may even make matters worse by further assaulting the beleaguered ecosystem and delaying proper treatment. *(See "The Lowdown on Nonprescription Yeast Treatments," page 128.)*

Yeast Infections

Unlike other types of vaginitis, yeast infections are caused not by a bacteria but by an overgrowth of one of several types of fungi called candida. The result: an odorless white, cottage cheese–like discharge and itching. A yeast infection will probably afflict you at least once during your lifetime, induced by a course of antibiotics, steroids, birth control pills, obesity, diabetes, pregnancy, or wearing fabrics that trap heat and moisture, such as nylon.

Yeast infections are combated with tablets or vaginal creams and suppositories, some of which are now available over the counter. When using a cream or suppository, wear a sanitary napkin to protect your clothes, and change pads frequently. You should wear cotton underwear and avoid panty hose to reduce moisture. Continue using the drug even during your menstrual period.

Doctors advise using OTC yeast treatments only if you've been recently diagnosed with a yeast infection and the exact same symptoms return—assuming you have not had a new sexual partner who might have introduced a new infectious agent. If you do buy a nonprescription yeast cream, look for those containing the active agents miconazole, butoconazole, or clotrimazole. (Beware that many yeast creams contain small amounts of oil, which can erode the latex in condoms and diaphragms, thus compromising these forms of birth control.)

Eating yogurt or taking acidophilus tablets to treat a yeast infection are controversial strategies. According to Hillier, this approach is "good theory, bad practice. The lactobacilli in yogurt and acidophilus are cousins to those in the vagina, but they're not the same strain and they won't help recolonize the vagina." However, an Israeli investigation conducted in 1996 showed that yogurt containing *lactobacillus acidophilus* reduced the incidence of both yeast infections and BV in women who regularly consumed it. It's safe to say that eating yogurt with live and active cultures as a preventive measure can't hurt you.

Caution: Yeast infections are considered a marker for HIV infection. If you have recurrent yeast infections and have had unprotected sex, you should get an HIV test.

Trichomoniasis

The third most common infection, trichomoniasis is a single-cell parasite that is usually transmitted during sex. (Wet towels, washcloths, and bathing suits are also occasionally the agents of infection.) The symptoms are an increased discharge that is frothy, yellow-green in color, and has a fishy odor. Itching, soreness, and painful urination and intercourse are often present as well.

As with bacterial vaginosis, there are possible health consequences if the infection is not treated. These include a greater risk for premature birth and low-birth-weight babies. The treatment of choice is the drug metronidazole. As with all antibiotics, avoid drinking alcohol until twenty-four hours after treatment is completed. It is critical to have your partner treated also, since reinfection is common.

COMMON VAGINAL INFECTIONS

Infection	Symptoms
Bacterial Vaginosis	Itching; foul, fishy odor; thin gray-white or gray discharge
Yeast Infections	Itching, burning; white cottage cheese–like discharge; no odor
Trichomoniasis	Itching; foul, fishy odor; frothy yellow-green discharge

Douches and Don'ts

Douching is one of the rituals that mothers pass on to their daughters—along with negative messages about their bodies and sexuality. "As women, we are taught to consider the vagina a dirty place," says Sharon Hillier, M.D., director of Reproductive Infectious Disease Research at Magee–Women's Hospital at the University of Pittsburgh. "Not to wash out the vagina is to risk being not considered sexually attractive."

As many as 37 percent of women ages fourteen to forty-four douche regularly, according to a study by the National Survey of Family Growth. Douching not only has no medical benefits, but research shows it is actually harmful to women's health. Women who douche have a greater chance of contracting bacterial vaginosis, which has been linked to higher rates of preterm birth, pelvic inflammatory disease (PID), and several other ailments. Those who douche before a gynecological exam are more likely to remain undiagnosed because they wash away the evidence of infection before the exam. Douching has also been shown to be associated with ectopic pregnancy and impaired fertility.

Women spend $250 million a year on over-the-counter yeast treatments, and for many they represent responsible self-care. "OTC medications have made an important contribution to women's health," says Anita Nelson, M.D., associate professor of gynecology at the Harbor–UCLA Medical Center. "For women who are experienced with vaginal infections, it is a blessing."

Unfortunately these medications are frequently used for the wrong reasons. Many women use them where there is any unusual discharge, believing the problem must be yeast. But using yeast cures without knowing what your problem is, is a bad idea for two reasons:

- First, yeast remedies will not work on infections that are caused by bacteria, such as bacterial vaginosis, the most common vaginal infection. By treating yourself for a yeast infection, you delay getting the proper treatment for

Vexing Viruses

Viruses present altogether different threats to vaginal health. The most common types are herpes simplex virus (HSV) and human papilloma virus (HPV), which causes genital warts. Viruses take up permanent residence in your body, and there are as yet no cures, so you can only treat the symptoms. Like other vaginal infections, HPV and HSV can increase your susceptibility for acquiring other STDs, including HIV.

Rates of HSV and HPV infection have increased in the last twenty years or so. They are more of a problem today because of some major societal shifts. In the past, these viruses were primarily contracted nonsexually in infancy and childhood, when there were more kids in the household who had close personal contact, notes Peter Lynch, M.D., chairman of the Department of Dermatology at the University of California at Davis, a specialist in vulvar dermatology. Acquiring HSV or HPV in childhood confers a slight vaccination effect.

When adults contract the viruses, having no immunity against them, they wind up with a more severe infection. Contracting viral infections during pregnancy is a particular cause for concern. It is not the time to have a new sexual partner whose STD status you do not know.

Herpes Simplex Virus (HSV)

Improved treatments have made the itching and painful blistering of genital herpes a little easier to live with in recent years. "Herpes has become more of a nuisance than a scarlet letter," says James MacGregor, M.D. As many as 20 percent of women have antibodies to the virus, meaning they've been exposed to it, but only about 5 percent will ever experience an outbreak. The first outbreak is usually the worst; subsequent episodes are briefer and less intense.

It's possible to get or give herpes even in the absence of the telltale blisters, so you should always include HSV when checking a new partner's STD status. Condoms will not completely protect an infected partner since the lesions can occur on the skin around the genital area. Antiviral drugs, including a newly approved medication called famciclovir, can help reduce outbreaks and the rate of unsymptomatic shedding, when someone who is infected "sheds" the virus in the absence of herpes blisters, thus protecting the one you love. Famciclovir has been shown to be more effective than the standard therapy, acyclovir, even in less frequent doses. More hope could come from the work of scientists exploring herpes vaccines, which would be particularly useful to couples in which only one partner was infected.

Acquiring the infection during pregnancy is particularly dangerous, since it is associated with a greater risk of miscarriage, certain pregnancy complications, preterm birth, and congenital infections. Today, doctors often treat infected pregnant women with antiviral agents through the pregnancy and birth, and deliver the baby by Cesarean section to avoid vaginal contact.

Human Papilloma Virus (HPV)

HPV refers to some eighty different viruses that are responsible for genital warts in and around the vagina. They sometimes itch and or burn after intercourse, but the greater danger is HPV's link to cervical cancer (see Chapter 2, page 14).

Not all types of HPV cause warts, however, and these types are actually more worrisome, because research indicates that they may be associated with cervical cancer. This may be good news for those who have visible warts, but it presents some treatment dilemmas. In the past practitioners removed the warts as a matter of course, using a variety of methods, ranging from cryotherapy (freezing) and topical drug treatments (podofilox, podophyllin) to laser or surgical removal, depending on their size and location. The warts often recur, however, and even if they don't, you can still infect your partner.

Some doctors believe that removing warts diminishes the chance that they will increase in size and number. Others say removal presents problems of its own: pain and scarring. And there's always a chance that the warts will disappear on their own.

If warts are painful or embarrassing to you, you may decide to have them removed. Your provider can help you review the treatment options.

Like herpes, some 20 percent of women have acquired HPV, though only 5 percent develop the bothersome warts associated with it. (For more information on HPV, see Chapter 7, page 166.)

When Love Hurts

Painful sex is sometimes a symptom of another complaint, such as endometriosis, fibroids, or pelvic inflammatory disease (see Chapter 2, page

the real source of your vaginal complaints, possibly increasing your risk for long-term health problems like pelvic inflammatory disease.

- Second, many women seeking treatment have more than one infection. So even if you do have a yeast infection, you may have a second bug that also needs attention.

The bottom line: If you have itching or irritation and an unnatural discharge, you need to be examined by a health-care provider who can determine the cause of your suffering. "A clinician cannot make a diagnosis without looking at a sample of your discharge under a microscope," says David E. Soper, M.D., director of the Division of Benign Gynecology at the Medical University of South Carolina. "Anything short of that is pure guesswork."

If you are diagnosed with a yeast infection and the same symptoms (white cottage cheese–like discharge, itching, and redness) return, an OTC product is appropriate—assuming you have not had new sexual partners since you were treated. If the symptoms differ from the ones you experienced with the diagnosed yeast infection, you need to be reexamined.

If you use an over-the-counter yeast treatment, be aware that some products marketed as yeast cures are not effective. Make sure the product you choose contains one of these ingredients: miconazole, butoconazole, or clotrimazole; some that do include Monistat, Femstat, and Gynelotrimin.

35). Other times, it is the primary problem. Here are some common vaginal culprits and their cures:

Vaginal Dryness

It's a fact of aging: "After menopause, 99 percent of women will experience vaginal dryness," says Geoffrey Redmond, M.D., an Ohio endocrinologist and author of *The Good News About Women's Hormones*. When the ovaries lose the ability to produce estrogen, the vagina gets drier. Natural moisture tapers off over time, increasing irritation and painful sex a few years after the end of menstruation.

According to Redmond, estrogen replacement, delivered in oral form like Premarin and Estrace, skin patches, and vaginal creams, is a superb solution—but it's important to get the optimal dose. "The minimal dose women get provides protection against heart disease and osteoporosis," he says, "but for most women these doses do not adequately relieve thin, dry tissue." Many women are embarrassed to bring up this seemingly frivolous problem, or they don't realize that an altered dose could help them. A good health-care provider can help you monitor your dose to avoid unwanted side effects and still get the relief you need to feel comfortable—and sexual. Providing your physician with feedback is the only way to help him fine-tune your treatment.

There are other options in the quick-fix category. The feminine products section at the drugstore now displays a dizzying array of slippery substances designed to keep your love life gliding happily along including vaginal moisturizers, jellies, and lubricants like Vagisil and Astroglide. (Always make sure that the lubricating substance you use is water soluble. Oil-based products can harm the vaginal ecosystem and erode the latex used in condoms.)

These products can also be useful to premenopausal women who experience dryness due to hysterectomy, childbirth, or nursing, and the absence of menstrual periods. The use of condoms or diaphragms, stress, excessive exercise, chemotherapy, some medications (antidepressants, antihistamines, and oral contraceptives), and various medical conditions like diabetes and multiple sclerosis can all cause vaginal dryness. There is another offbeat solution: the female condom, brand-named Reality. Some menopausal women have taken to using it with a lubricant to protect thinning tissues from potential damage from intercourse because the condom stays motionless relative to the walls of the vagina.

Vulvodynia

Painful intercourse sometimes has other, more mysterious, causes. Tops on this list is vulvodynia, which is not really a disease itself but a set of symptoms—burning, rawness, stinging, or irritation of the vulva and vaginal opening—for which the cause is not known.

Unfortunately most doctors are ill equipped to deal with the complaint. Gynecologists are trained to deal with reproductive health problems, while dermatologists are largely unfamiliar with gynecological disorders that may affect the vulvar area. "Dermatologists are not trained to evaluate the vagina," says Libby Edwards, M.D., a vulvar specialist with the Carolinas Medical Center in Charlotte, North Carolina. As a result, when women turn up with unusual vulvar symptoms, their complaints may be dismissed or minimized.

The source of the discomfort is often inflammation of the nerves or a skin problem, but vulvodynia can also stem from a complication of herpes simplex, an unusually stubborn strain of yeast, abnormal vaginal discharge, low estrogen levels, or concentration of a chemical called oxalate in the urine. It does not have a psychological basis, although it can lead to depression since the discomfort is often chronic and unremitting.

Sex under these conditions is painful—if not impossible—and profoundly upsetting. "It affects a woman in ways that strike at her self-esteem and feelings of femininity," says Edwards. "When you are in pain, you lose interest in sex. You become angry and resentful of your partner for wanting it. Then you feel guilty."

There is no simple test for vulvodynia, so doctors tend to treat a woman's symptoms through trial and error. Doctors often try amitriptyline or desipramine, two antidepressants now widely prescribed for nerve-related pain. Some women find relief by following a diet that is low in oxalate and by taking calcium citrate, which may help excrete oxalate. Other approaches: cortisone ointments and even biofeedback.

Vulvodynia finally received some recognition in April 1997 when the National Institutes of Health convened a symposium on the mysterious ailment. The meeting gave dermatologists, gynecologists, and neurologists an opportunity to put their heads together and swap information, theories, and treatment strategies.

If you have symptoms that sound like vulvodynia, and your doctor seems unable to help you or suggests that the problem is all in your head, contact the National Vulvodynia Association (301-299-0775). The association disseminates information about the ailment and puts women in touch with local support networks.

Foods High in Oxalate

beans (dried)	black pepper
beer	celery
beets	chocolate
berries	citrus peel
berry juices	cocoa
collards	pecans
concord grapes	rhubarb
eggplant	spinach
escarole	summer squash
fruit cake	sweet potatoes
green peppers	tangerines
grits	tea
kale	tofu
mustard greens	watercress
leeks	wheat germ
peanuts	

Vaginismus

Unlike vulvodynia, vaginismus—which is an involuntary spasm of the vaginal muscles that causes pain and sometimes makes penetration impossible—does have psychological roots. The problem is often related to a previous experience such as sexual abuse or to an irrational fear or anxiety about sex. "Vaginismus is the body's way of protecting a woman against some terror," says Anita Nelson, M.D.

If a woman has experienced painful intercourse stemming from a physical cause like endometriosis, she may also develop vaginismus because she begins to anticipate pain during sex. This form of the disorder is called secondary vaginismus.

The extent of vaginismus can range widely—some women find even the insertion of a tampon excruciating, while others can manage medical procedures but are unable to have sexual intercourse. The first step is to rule out anatomical defects, such as a wall of tissue that may have developed unnaturally from birth, causing searing pain with penetration.

Treatment often includes:

- *Dilating the vaginal muscles*. Dilators come in graduated sizes and are used progressively until the woman is able to relax her muscles with insertion. Once the muscles relax, she advances to the next larger size.
- *Muscle-awareness exercises*. Such exercises teach women to contract their muscles and therefore understand the difference between contracted and relaxed muscles.
- *Counseling*. Psychotherapy (or other types of counseling) is often a necessary adjunct to these physical therapies.

Vestibulitis

Vestibulitis is an inflammation at the opening of the vagina that causes extreme pain during penetration. Human papilloma virus as well as chemical irritants—soaps, bubble bath, even fabric softener—are sometimes to blame. Vestibulitis is not an infection, so antibiotics are not likely to work. Hydrocortisone and estrogen creams do a better job. Discuss the problem with your doctor to determine the cause and course of treatment.

Pain with Orgasm

This rare condition is literally the agony and the ecstasy. Just as a woman climaxes, she experiences excruciating pain, followed by soreness. Although no one knows what causes the condition, it is easily treated by taking anti-inflammatory pain killers such as ibuprofen prior to intercourse.

Retroverted Uterus

Between 15 and 30 percent of women have what is called a retroverted uterus. Most of them have no sexual complications, but a few experience pain when the penis comes into contact with the uterus or ovaries during deep thrusting. If you have a retroverted uterus, you may wish to experiment with different sexual positions until you find one that is comfortable. Being on top helps you control the angle and depth of penetration.

Bartholin's Gland Cysts

The Bartholin's glands, located just inside the vagina, secrete fluid during sexual arousal. When the gland becomes clogged by an infection, a cyst may form, causing pain, irritation, and redness at the vaginal opening, especially if the gland becomes abscessed. The treatment: opening the area and allowing the cyst to drain. In serious cases, a catheter may be inserted for several days to keep the cyst draining.

Burning Love: Urinary Tract Infections

You're basking in the glow of a new romance—one that's been heating up things in your bedroom for several days running. Just when you think there's no end to your bliss, you find yourself suddenly and urgently needing to urinate. When you do, it stings, burns, and hurts. The honeymoon is over—at least temporarily.

If you are sexually active and haven't joined the cystitis club yet, you probably will. It's a big group, comprised mostly of women. Cystitis, also known as a urinary tract infection (UTI), strikes women twenty-five times more often than men and accounts for some 5 million doctor visits a year. It is especially common during pregnancy.

While UTIs are not associated with sex in every case, sexual practices are often to blame in one way or another. Any time bacteria—especially the ubiquitous E. coli—find their way to your urethra, they can easily travel into the bladder, where they flourish and eventually trigger the symptoms of infection.

The intimate contact of sex itself provides a perfect conduit because bacteria from women's bodies and their partners' bodies is pushed into the vagina. Recent data have also shown that some sex-related behaviors, such as the use of spermicides containing nonoxynol-9, can increase your risk for a UTI, probably by altering the vaginal flora and increasing the pool of infection-causing bugs in your vagina. The same mechanism may be at work with diaphragms, which have long been thought to promote infection by putting pressure on the bladder or urethra. This was believed to cause bacteria to back up into the bladder. Some experts now think that the spermicides used with diaphragms contribute to the problem. Research shows that spermicide-coated condoms may also alter the vaginal ecology, leading to an increased risk for urinary tract infections, according to Stephan D. Fihn, M.D., director of the Health Services Research Program at the Seattle (Washington) Veterans Affairs Medical Center.

There's also evidence that women may be more likely to come down with cystitis after a visit to the gynecologist, according to Jeffrey D. Tiemstra, M.D., director of the Department of Family Medicine at the University of Illinois College of Medicine in Urbana. Bacteria is probably pushed into the urinary tract during the pelvic exam. But drinking water and urinating after your exam will minimize the risk of getting an infection, Tiemstra says, "certainly if you are someone who has had trouble with infections in the past."

There are lots of myths about UTIs. Some have turned out to be false;

others have withstood the scrutiny of modern research. Cranberry juice, a decades-old home remedy, does indeed reduce the rate of recurring infections. It apparently contains chemicals that prevent bacteria from sticking to the urethra and bladder. Blueberries contain the same chemicals.

On the other hand, the notion of wiping from front to back after using the toilet as a way to prevent UTIs may have no basis. "The idea of 'wiping wrong' has been dispelled for a few years now," says Alice Stellenwork Petrulis, M.D., associate professor of medicine and reproductive biology at Case Western Reserve University in Cleveland. Wiping from front to back may prevent other infections, however.

Whatever the cause, there are increasingly effective treatments and some solid strategies for keeping your love life on track and preventing the recurrence of cystitis.

The symptoms: Burning and stinging when urinating, increased frequency and urgency of urination, often blood in the urine, and pain. Symptoms of infection often occur twelve to twenty-four hours after sexual intercourse.

The solution: Your health-care provider may want to test you before treatment to find out what bacteria is responsible for the infection so as to prescribe the right antibiotic. Otherwise she will probably put you on a broad-spectrum drug, which targets more than one type of bacteria, so as to get you out of your misery as soon as possible. Always take the entire course of antibiotics. You don't want to run the risk of having the infection return in a more severe form.

Providers have successfully treated cystitis with briefer and briefer doses of antibiotics. Treatment for UTIs used to involve taking a drug for fourteen days. This often had the effect of triggering yeast infections by disrupting the vaginal ecology. Today the standard treatment period is three to five days, though some clinicians have experimented with regimens of even shorter duration. "One-dose regimens are not as in vogue as they were a few years ago because they have a slightly higher recurrence rate," says Tamara Bavendam, M.D., director of the Center for Pelvic Floor Disorders at Allegheny University of the Health Sciences in Philadelphia.

Women prone to recurring infections are sometimes treated with low daily doses of antibiotics taken over a period of time to prevent infection. And doctors are experimenting with new methods of self-treatment for

SEXUAL HYGIENE

How can you keep cystitis from wrecking your sex life? Tamara Bavendam, M.D., director of the Center for Pelvic Floor Disorders at Allegheny University of the Health Sciences in Philadelphia, offers these suggestions:

- Clean yourself before and after sex to keep the genital area clear of harmful bacteria. "You don't have to be religious, just use common sense," Bavendam says.
- Urinate immediately after sex to head off any bacteria that have made their way into the bladder. If you must urinate beforehand, drink a glass of water then so that you'll need to empty your bladder again afterward. "What's important is urinating afterward with a good volume," she says.
- If you first have anal intercourse, make sure your partner washes his penis thoroughly before entering your vagina. The rectum is a prime source of E. coli, the bacteria implicated in many UTIs.

such women. Doctors may prescribe antibiotics for these women to keep on hand and use for a few days when symptoms flare.

While you're waiting for the drug to kick in, try these things to soothe symptoms:

- Sit in a warm tub. Just don't add any bubble bath, bath oils, or other chemicals that can further irritate the urethra.
- Two drugs, phenazopyridine hydrochloride (Pyridium) and methenamine (Prosed, Urised), are known to relieve urinary discomfort. Be warned: They turn your urine bright red and blue, respectively. (If you're in a bind and can't reach someone who can call in a prescription for you, ask the pharmacist about over-the-counter versions of phenazopyridine hydrochloride.)

There's also a new over-the-counter test kit for UTIs (called UTI), which indicates the presence of the most common UTI-related bacteria. It comes with six urine collection cups and test strips. The kit provides a good way for women to confirm whether early symptoms are associated with a bacterial invasion that a doctor should treat. (Your provider will still have to test you to determine the type of bacteria you have so as to prescribe the appropriate antibiotic.) The kit also allows women with recurrent infections to monitor the effectiveness of their antibiotic regimen.

When It's Not a UTI

Sometimes what seems like a UTI is not an infection at all. There's a feeling of urgency and burning with urination, but when you're tested for bacteria, there's nothing abnormal in your urine.

This so-called hypersensitivity syndrome afflicts a minority of women, and for them UTI treatments are often inappropriate. The bladder may actually be irritated by the acidity in cranberry juice, for example. "Cranberry juice is not a cure-all for all bladder problems," Bavendam says.

For such women, drinking water with a small amount of baking soda mixed in may offer relief. For others, calcium tablets like Tums or Rolaids will do the trick. Some people believe that such dietary changes as avoiding citrus fruits, spicy foods, onions, vegetable fats, and chocolate may make a difference, too.

Burning Bladder Syndromes

At the extreme of sensitive bladder problems is a rare disorder known as interstitial cystitis, in which the bladder wall is sensitive and feels full. Treatments include a drug that must be inserted by catheter into the bladder or a procedure that physically stretches it. The first oral drug for interstitial cystitis, called Elmiron, was introduced to the market in 1996. It is reported to relieve symptoms in 40 percent of patients who use it.

A similar problem is urethral diverticulum, a defect in the urethral "tube" that may produce a variety of symptoms, from incontinence to infection to painful intercourse.

Love Is a Contact Sport: Sex Injuries

Caution: Sex involves some very sensitive body parts, and intimacy can sometimes lead to serious injury. Here's what you should know before you hit the sheets.

Hers

Because of their sexual anatomy, women tend to sustain more injuries during sex than men, including bruises and even tears in the vaginal wall due to overly enthusiastic partners. Injuries are most common in women in their twenties, though postmenopausal women may be more biologically vulnerable because the vaginal walls become thinner and drier due to the lack of estrogen. (Sex injuries are common among victims of sexual assaults.) Deep thrusting can cause pain to the ovaries, usually a sharp, sudden pain. It's similar in severity to the pain a man experiences after being kicked in the groin.

His

Intercourse can also harm a man's sexual anatomy, and the erect penis is a particularly vulnerable organ. Technically speaking, the penis is actually a pair of chambers that fill with fluid during sexual arousal, like balloons. They are covered by a protective covering called the tunica. Too much pressure in the wrong place can do serious damage.

The most dramatic injury is a penile fracture or *faux pas au coit*. It happens most frequently with a misplaced thrust into a woman's pubic bone, the area between her vagina and anus, or even the mattress. The blow creates undue pressure in the penile chambers, causing blood to burst through the tunica. The result: a cracking sound, followed by swelling and bruising. Immediate attention is required because untreated fractures can lead to impotence.

Bent penis, or Peyronie's disease, results from the same bungles in bed, but it is less serious. It happens when the tunica sustains a blow that scratches it. As the injury tries to heal, the scratch gets stretched over

- The day after sex, drink plenty of fluids (at least six to eight glasses) and urinate frequently to keep the bladder flushed. "You want dilute urine, which is lighter in color. If urine is concentrated (dark yellow), you need to drink more."
- In general, drink fluids in abundance and try to urinate at least every three to four hours. Don't hold it in. It's also important not to urinate too frequently because going when you don't really need to is a way of training your bladder to become smaller.

The best way to deal with sex injuries is to avoid them in the first place. Communicating about what is comfortable is your first line of defense. The woman-on-top position will give you more control over where your partner's penis goes. (By the same token, the male-superior position gives him more control.) A few more sex safety tips:

For women:

- If you feel any pain during intercourse, speak up and change positions.
- If pain continues over time, it might signal an underlying problem like endometriosis or fibroids. Schedule a visit with your health-care provider.
- If sexual friction is irritating, try a lubricant (Astroglide, Vagisil). Too much friction makes mishaps more likely. (If vaginal dryness is a chronic problem, consult a physician.)
- Use extra caution during deep or energetic thrusting.

time by a man's regular nocturnal erections. The penis bends at the point of the injury. For most men, Peyronie's causes only a slight bending that does not interfere with sex. Men with more severe bends may experience pain and find intercourse difficult. Treatments include vitamin E, which diminishes the scarring, a drug called Potaba, steroid injections or, in the most serious cases, surgery.

Another common male sex injury is priapism, a prolonged, painful erection that may result from vigorous and sustained sex. (Priapism can also be caused by sickle-cell anemia, leukemia, neurologic disorders, and certain medications.) Impotence can result if the condition is not treated promptly by a doctor. Drugs will often ease the erection, but if they do not, a needle is inserted into the penis to release the buildup of fluid.

Losing That Loving Feeling: Sexual Dysfunction

Orgasm disorders afflict some 30 percent of women in Europe and the United States, and sexual desire problems affect another 20 percent. But many women choose to suffer in silence when their bodies betray them in bed. Sexual problems—from unresolved emotional issues to the side effects of aging—tend to go underground. This echoes women's reactions to many other issues relating to sexual anatomy and function.

Addressing these problems involves untangling a complex web of physical, psychological, and cultural factors. Fortunately these factors are increasingly the focus of medical interest.

Prescription for Problems

Even without the rock 'n' roll, sex and drugs can be a risky mix, threatening a woman's interest in sex or her ability to enjoy its pleasures. Numerous medications can sabotage sexual functioning by inhibiting desire, lowering libido, or interfering with orgasm. An article in *The Journal of Family Practice* listed more than 150 over-the-counter, prescription, and illicit drugs that may impair sex. From migraine and stomach medications to antibiotics and OTC antihistamines, these are the drugs of daily life—the kind our pill-popping generation doesn't think twice about taking.

Unfortunately, sexual side effects are rarely discussed when a doctor hands a patient a prescription. For starters, both doctors and patients are notorious for clamming up when it comes to sex-related issues. More often, physicians just plain don't know that the prescribed drug may have sexual side effects. The *Physician's Desk Reference*, the drug bible that describes drug mechanisms and interactions, rarely mentions sexual side effects. "The *PDR* is sexually dysfunctional," claims Theresa Crenshaw, M.D., a San Diego sex therapist and author of *Sexual Pharmacology*.

But even when doctors are aware of a drug's potential for undermining intimacy, they may not clue their patients in because they think the information itself might trigger sexual difficulties. "They fear a self-fulfilling prophecy," Crenshaw says. "It's naive but well intended." To make matters worse, sexual drug reactions often surface gradually, even months after a patient has gone on a new drug, reducing the chance that she will connect the problem to the prescription. This information gap can set the stage for long-term sexual woes—especially for younger women who have yet to discover their sexual patterns.

Many women would be surprised to learn that their sexual problems might be due to the progesterone in their oral contraceptives. Progesterone is considered antiandrogenic, meaning it reduces the body's testosterone levels. In some women this has the effect of diminishing sex drive or delaying orgasm. In some cases physicians can skirt the problem by substituting a different pill with a higher dose of estrogen in relation to its progesterone, suggests David Pang, M.D., a spokesperson for the American Association of Pharmaceutical Scientists.

But this is not an option with birth control methods that contain progesterone only, such as mini-pills, Norplant, and Depo-Provera. "This is one of the most obvious areas where there's really no excuse for doctors not to alert their patients," Crenshaw says. No one knows how many women lose their libido to progesterone, but their ranks could be substantial considering how many women are on the hormone, including postmenopausal women taking hormone replacement therapy. (Ironically, preserving sex drive is a top research priority with scientists who are developing a male Pill.)

Sexual problems are a well-known—and well-studied—phenomenon with the new class of antidepressants known as selective serotonin reuptake inhibitors (or SSRIs), including Prozac, Zoloft, and Paxil. As women are twice as likely to suffer from depression, they are more often the victims of these drugs' libido-busting effects. And in a study published in a 1997 issue of the journal *Clinical Pharmacology and Therapeutics*, researchers reported the number of people on SSRIs who have adverse sexual effects may be far higher than reported previously—nearly three quarters of them experienced lowered libido, a lack of arousal, a delay in

For men:

- Never force an erect penis into clothing or slap it to turn off an erection.
- Be careful about the angle of penetration.
- Seek prompt medical attention if you hear any popping or cracking sounds or you experience pain during intercourse.

WHEN ANTIDEPRES-
SANTS DEPRESS YOUR
LOVE LIFE

Depression takes a toll on the body and the mind, but the cure may also carry a price. While antidepressants like Prozac or Zoloft—called selective serotonin reuptake inhibitors (SSRIs)—may lift patients' moods, these increasingly popular medications may also produce sexual side effects, from loss of desire to insufficient lubrication.

Many doctors can now offer a solution: weekend "drug holidays." In studies, Anthony Rothschild, M.D., a psychiatrist at the Harvard Medical School, found that patients on Paxil and Zoloft enjoyed a respite from their sexual symptoms—while their moods remained stable—when they took a three-day break from their drugs. This strategy, however, did not work for Prozac, which takes longer to leave the body.

Patients in the study stopped taking their medication on Thursday morning and resumed it again on Sunday night for a period of

orgasm, or a reduction in orgasmic intensity. (See "When Antidepressants Depress Your Love Life," left.)

Unwanted sexual side effects like desire and orgasm disorders can plague patients on the ulcer drug Tagamet. The problem also applies to its reduced-dose cousin Tagamet HB, which recently leaped over the counter—and into a greater number of medicine cabinets—as a heartburn remedy. Fortunately there are alternative ulcer and heartburn medicines, such as carafate, that are less likely to produce troublesome sexual side effects. More important, many ulcers do not require long-term drug treatment because they are caused by a bacteria that can be banished with only a brief course of antibiotics.

Sedatives and tranquilizers can also cause unpleasant sexual surprises, and women receive 80 percent of the prescriptions for such drugs. The biggest offenders: the benzodiazepines, which include Xanax, Valium, and Ativan. These medications suppress the central nervous system and thus may reduce sexual desire and response. And of course any drug that puts you to sleep, such as Halcion, can also do the same to your sex life.

Other drugs that can wreak havoc on a woman's sex life: Danazol, a male hormone that is used to counter endometriosis and fibrocystic breast disease, and Inderal, a migraine medication. And antibiotics can trigger yeast infections—something you can count on to dampen your love life.

Even nonprescription drugs can produce problems in bed. Potential sex stoppers include over-the-counter antihistamines like Benadryl and sleeping pills like Nytol and Sominex, which rely on the same active ingredient, diphenhydramine. These drugs may interfere with the ability to reach orgasm. Antihistamines and decongestants can also contribute to vaginal irritation and painful sex by drying out the body's mucus membranes. (Women who use them regularly may find relief with artificial vaginal lubricants.)

Sexual side effects are serious issues, not simply nuisances that go away when drug treatment ends. In fact, they can set up lifelong sexual problems. "Women are placed on 'sex offender' drugs like antidepressants, tranquilizers, and birth control pills in their twenties and thirties before they've even established their own sexual patterns," says Crenshaw. "By the time they're taken off the drugs, they feel so sexually dysfunctional that often they remain dysfunctional."

What to do? First, read the packaging for any drug you are prescribed. "If the package insert says: 'Do not drive or operate a moving vehicle,' it's probably going to have some mild to severe impact on your sex life,"

Crenshaw says. (The warning is a tip-off that the drug affects the central nervous system and may interfere with the mechanisms of arousal and orgasm.)

It's embarrassing to talk about sexual side effects with a doctor, but doing so can save you considerable grief in the future. Don't hesitate to mention *Sexual Pharmacology,* a drug reference published in 1996 that lists the drug mechanisms that can help a physician interpret the *PDR* to determine if a medication might threaten sex.

Sometimes altering the dosage or the timing of a drug can reduce its side effects without diminishing its effectiveness. And if changing the dose doesn't work, there are often appropriate alternatives. But stopping or altering the dose of a medication is risky business and should only be undertaken with the guidance of a physician.

A Note About Recreational Drugs and Sex

A host of recreational and illicit drugs can interfere with healthy sexual functioning. Among the recreational drugs with sexual side effects are alcohol, cocaine, barbiturates, amphetamines, marijuana, and Quaaludes. (See the following page for a complete list.)

The Gender Gap in Sex Research

Despite the high percentages of sex problems among females, little is known about the sexual process in women. Doctors are often in the dark, therefore, when it comes to diagnosing and treating female sexual woes.

"The research done over the last twenty years is exclusively in the domain of *male* sexual dysfunction," says Irwin Goldstein, M.D., a professor of urology at Boston University School of Medicine.

For instance, although few researchers have explored the physical problems that hinder sex in women, the sources of erectile dysfunction—the new and kinder name for impotence—have been exhaustively studied and catalogued. Doctors know that diabetes and vascular changes, along with many commonly prescribed medications, top the list of culprits and that psychological issues are involved in a small percentage of cases. While men now have a repertoire of physical remedies, women are simply sent to therapy.

According to Goldstein, however, there's every reason to think the factors that produce sexual problems in men can be pitfalls to women, too. "Blood flow plays a big role in orgasm. Hardening of the arteries, high cholesterol, cigarette smoking—all the things that can cause heart at-

four weeks. Because patients are usually on SSRIs for months at a time, researchers are now testing whether the regimen works over a longer period. "We want to find out if you can keep doing this and continue the drug's efficacy," Rothschild says. Again, altering the dosage of a drug is tricky business, so you should only do so under a physician's guidance.

Side effects can often be avoided by substituting another antidepressant. There's evidence that the new drug Wellbutrin can successfully treat the blues without sabotaging sex. (In some studies, it even heightened sexual function.) In addition, more people are turning to St. John's wort, an herbal depression remedy popular in Germany that appears to have no sexual side effects. Or doctors may prescribe other drugs that restore sexual response, such as yohimbine or cyproheptadine. In any case, your doctor should also rule out other causes of sexual dysfunction—including, of course, the depression itself.

141

tacks—also block the arteries of the penis, leading to impotence," he says. "In the past there was a belief that this phenomenon only exists in males and that the clitoris and vagina get perfect circulation. Women were told that problems were all in their mind."

Thankfully this is changing. Swept along with the surge of new interest in women's health research, female sexual processes are beginning to get some attention in research labs. Goldstein, for instance, has created a new model for female sexual dysfunction by deliberately clogging the arteries in female rats. The resulting reduction in blood flow diminished sexual response and function. Goldstein has identified two distinct conditions, "vaginal engorgement insufficiency syndrome" and "clitoral erectile insufficiency syndrome," both the products of the inflicted vascular changes. Both conditions could explain a woman's inability to become sexually stimulated.

PHARMACEUTICAL SEX STOPPERS

Here are some of the drugs that may affect sex drive and function:

Antianxiety: Klonopin, Librium, Valium, Xanax, Ativan

Antiarrhythmics (for heart irregularities): Lanoxin, Mexitil, Norpace, Procan

Antidepressants: Ascendin, Elavil, Nardil, Paxil, Prozac, Sinequan, Tofranil, Zoloft

Anticonvulsants: Dilantin, Tegretol

Antihistamines: Atarax, Benadryl, Chlor-Trimeton

Antihypertensives: Catapres, Inderal, Lopressor, Procardia, Timoptic

Anti-Infectives: Mexate, Nizoral, Septra, Virazole

Antipsychotics: Haldol, Mellaril, Prolixin, Thorazine

Gastrointestinal drugs: Reglen, Tagamet

Diuretics: Aldactone, Hydrodiuril, Hygroton

Hormones: Megace, oral contraceptives, Prednisone, Provera

Muscle relaxant: Lioresal

Sleeping medications: Halcion, Phenobarbitol, Restoril; or *over-the-counter:* Nytol, Unisom, Sominex, Sleep-Eze

Headache medications: Inderal

Sources: *The Kinsey Institute New Report on Sex* (New York: St. Martin's Press, 1990) and *Sexual Pharmacology* (New York: W. W. Norton, 1996).

Other researchers are mapping the complex biochemical mechanisms of arousal and orgasm and checking out the psychological cofactors of sexual dysfunction in women. "We're playing catch-up," Goldstein says. This work is yielding some new sexual strategies for female intimacy problems (see "Jump-Starting Sex: A New Sex Therapy for Women," page 151), and Goldstein predicts the work will lead to the development of new drugs. These sex-fix pills would target specific biochemical processes involved in sex for both men and women. The drug Viagra, for instance, recently approved for the treatment of male sexual dysfunction, may prove helpful to women, too.

The Thrill Is Gone: Lack of Libido

How could something so good go so wrong? This is not the latest cry-in-your-beer honky-tonk hit but the silent refrain of millions of couples across America. Desire disorders affect some 15 million American women and rank among the top reasons that people seek sex counseling.

Domeena C. Renshaw, M.D., director of the Loyola Sexual Dysfunction Clinic in Maywood, Illinois, refers to loss of libido as "sexual anorexia nervosa"—after the eating disorder that's marked by an extreme avoidance of food. As with eating disorders, women are more apt to be the victims of desire problems—not surprising when you consider all the things that can come between them and bliss in bed:

- Body-image issues—the bane of many a woman's existence—are magnified during sex. Unrealistic ideals keep many women from abandoning themselves to erotic feelings or sexual pleasure. A loving, supportive partner and counseling can help. (See "Body Image and Sexuality," page 145.)
- Negative cultural attitudes toward sex hit women hard. "We teach little girls that genitals are dirty," says Anita Nelson, M.D., associate professor of obstetrics and gynecology at the Harbor–UCLA Medical Center. "But then they're also expected to be sex kittens."
- Women, bearing most of the birth control burden and most of the consequences of its potential failure, are more prone to contraceptive worries that sink the desire for sex. Choosing a method that is right for you and optimizing its effectiveness can go a long way toward restoring your interest in intimacy. (See Chapter 4, "Contraceptive Consciousness," page 49.)
- Concerns about contracting a sexually transmitted disease can also sidetrack sex. It's important to learn how to protect yourself with

safe-sex practices and discover ways of getting your partner to co-operate. (*See Chapter 7, "The Scourges of Love: Sexually Transmitted Diseases," page 157.*)

- Women who suffer from uncomfortable or painful intercourse may lose the desire for sex because they associate it with pain. If painful sex is a problem, discuss the problem with your health-care provider and seek treatment—for the sake of both your health and your love life.

- Many diseases and chronic health conditions, such as arthritis, inhibit sexual interest. Though temporary illnesses rarely lead to permanent sexual problems, libido lapses stemming from a long-term ailment may call for new sexual strategies that are satisfying to both partners.

- Menopause often triggers dips in desire due to shifting hormones and physical problems like vaginal dryness. The problem can frequently be reversed through hormone replacement therapy or through alternative remedies such as testosterone replacement. (*See "Hormone Therapy: The Debate Continues," page 189.*)

- Intimacy problems often show up as side effects of clinical depression, particularly in cases involving past sexual abuse. Recognizing and dealing with these problems is essential to sexual health.

- Declines in desire are a natural part of a relationship's ups and downs. Unresolved anger or a crisis in the relationship like a partner's infidelity are sure to trigger erotic apathy. They almost always call for couples counseling.

Lifestyle Lust Busters

Stress, fatigue, and boredom are the common colds of sexual dysfunction—they are such routine libido busters they border on cliché. According to Anita Nelson, M.D., associate professor of gynecology at the Harbor–UCLA Medical Center, the modern-day dance to balance work, family, and social commitments is simply incompatible with sexual spontaneity.

"There's the whole element of distraction. As you're doing one thing, you're thinking about the next. It's part of what makes us successful in the world," Nelson says. "But it doesn't work with sex." In other words, if you're thinking about work or wondering whether you put the clothes in the dryer, you're probably not connecting with your partner or tending to your own needs for intimacy.

Being too busy or too stressed may be common excuses for sexual indifference, but they should not be taken lightly. There are solid strategies for jump-starting sex even when counseling is not an option. Nelson's suggestions: Plan sexual surprises or experiment with new positions, places, and provocations—whatever it takes to keep you in the here-and-now.

Body Image and Sexuality

Whether they are responding to cultural forces or the pull of their own human nature, women feel the pressure to measure up to a feminine ideal. Women have had their feet bound, their ribs removed, and their skin pierced, all to fulfill a culture's vision of what it means to be beautiful.

America's cosmetic and fashion industries make billions exploiting this need. Each year nearly half a million women risk their health with cosmetic surgical procedures intended to correct their outward "imperfections"—small breasts, plain or unusual facial features, or excess fat. Eating disorders are epidemic among adolescent girls, and increasing numbers of older women binge and purge or starve themselves in a painful quest to ensure their attractiveness to others.

Whether or not they go to such extremes, women tend to have a volatile relationship with their bodies and this has obvious repercussions on their sexual well-being. How you feel about your body influences not only your choice of partners but your general attitude toward sex.

When *Shape* magazine explored the issue in its 1997 body image and sexuality survey, the editors were not surprised to learn that negative body attitudes adversely affect sexuality, but the outpouring from readers underscored how profound the issue is for many women.

"If I looked like I want to look, sex would be even greater because I wouldn't be so self-conscious," wrote one thirty-year-old reader. "I know my body image affects my love life," said another. "I feel embarrassed because I'm not skinny."

Many readers attached long letters to their questionnaires. The saddest of these came from women who blamed their unsatisfactory sex lives on their negative body image. "I have always felt that my poor body image holds me back sexually," one twenty-three-year-old wrote. "I have been dating the same guy for three years and although we have sex regularly (and safely, of course), I don't recall ever being comfortable. At 5 foot 5 and 145 pounds, I am a far cry from sexy. I can't allow myself to be free, wild, and crazy giving him the time of his life because I am too concerned with which of my bulges is in his way and how unvoluptuous my chest is."

Indeed the survey confirmed that many women harbor hang-ups about their body that may hinder their happiness in bed. The data showed that the women who were most unhappy with their bodies were those who reported being least comfortable having sex with the lights on and undressing in front of their partners. They were also the least likely to have orgasms during sex. Significantly they reported being least satisfied with themselves overall and generally the most self-conscious.

If your negative body image is affecting your sexuality, you are clearly not alone—but you can do something about it. Here are three things to help improve your body image and your intimate experiences:

1. *Get Acquainted with Your Body.* Get used to looking at your body in the mirror. The reason: Research shows that the part of body women are most comfortable with is the face. That's because they look at their faces more than any other body part. "Women need to spend more time getting to know their bodies again," says Anne Kearney-Cooke, Ph.D., director of the Cincinnati Psychotherapy Institute and an expert in body-image issues and eating disorders.

2. *Celebrate Your Body.* When you eat healthful foods and treat your body well, you are likely to feel better about it. Engaging in exercise triggers the same attitude adjustment. Consider the idea that you have a right to enjoy your body, not just to display it. That means learning to tune in to all your bodily senses. Savor foods, flavors, sights, and sounds. If you can learn to enjoy your body in other areas of your life, you can do it in bed.

3. *Reach Out and Touch Someone.* In general, develop more of a sensual self. Be deliberate about getting more touch in everyday life. Allow yourself to take pleasure in making physical contact with others, and touch others more. It's a self-reinforcing process: The more you touch, the more you feel like being touched.

Illness and Intimacy

When you come down with the flu, a romp in bed is the last thing on your mind. But libido is usually restored along with your good health.

But when the illness is very serious or a chronic medical condition, normal sexual expression may be profoundly altered.

Many illnesses, including cardiovascular disease, arthritis, urinary stress incontinence, and chronic pain, are themselves associated with sexual dysfunction. And illness can decrease your sexual self-esteem and sense of desirability. Many chronic conditions influence body image or may evoke negative responses from a partner.

Talking about sex with your physician when you are diagnosed can help ease your concerns about how your sex life will change and provide you with tools for solving problems if they arise. Certain positions, for instance, may make intercourse more comfortable for arthritis sufferers, and paraplegics can learn satisfying new ways to make love.

Breast cancer is one of the diseases most studied for its impact on a woman's life and sexuality. Since the breast is a focal point of sexual behavior and interest, mastectomy has obvious repercussions on a woman's sex life. Emotional problems during recovery often surround this challenge to her body image, as well.

Chemotherapy and radiation treatments can affect both sexual drive and functioning by drying the vagina. Vaginal dryness can be alleviated with estrogen creams or lubricants until normal moisture is restored. On the body-image front, women who seek reconstruction after mastectomy often experience a return to their normal, positive feelings. In fact, in one study, women who had undergone breast reconstruction were even more comfortable with their sexuality than they were before they were diagnosed with breast cancer.

Sex After Hysterectomy

When talking to a woman about the aftermath of hysterectomy, which involves the removal of the uterus and sometimes the ovaries and fallopian tubes, many doctors skimp on the sexual details. Women often don't think to ask. You have a right to know how the surgery may affect your interest in and capacity for the intimate behaviors you are used to experiencing.

In its technical bulletin on sexual dysfunction, the American College of Obstetricians and Gynecologists reports that hysterectomy typically shortens the vagina. Postmenopausal women are usually more affected by this change. The surgery can also change the position of the remaining organs, which shift around to fill the space. However, trying different sexual positions can help alleviate discomfort during intercourse (the woman-on-top position is a good place to start) and help partners find new sources of pleasurable sensations.

After the hysterectomy, orgasm itself often changes. This may be due in part to the loss of a hormone called prostacyclin, which is produced in the uterus. Women also cease to have uterine contractions, which can affect the intensity of their orgasms and may represent a major loss to a woman's sexuality.

Orgasm can also be affected by the removal of the cervix, which is a routine part of hysterectomy surgery. The cervix contains numerous nerves that may be stimulated during deep thrusting.

In some cases doctors may be able to perform cervix-sparing surgery, which may have less of an impact on sexual functioning. "Studies support the fact that if the cervix is left, women don't report a change in sexual response," says Beverly Whipple, Ph.D., an associate professor of nursing at Rutgers University in Newark, New Jersey.

When hysterectomy involves the removal of the ovaries, it produces changes that affect a woman's body in the same ways as menopause. Women may experience lowered libido and a lack of lubrication and dry, thinning tissue that make sex painful. Hormone replacement therapy can ease these symptoms, and a nonprescription lubricant can help with all but the libido. It's good to know that your capacity to have an orgasm should not change because sensation and arousal originate in the vagina and clitoris.

But hysterectomy can still diminish a woman's sense of her desirability and femininity, which may be harder to correct. It's important to realize that the loss of your reproductive capacity does not diminish your attractiveness to others or make you any less a woman.

Studies have shown the hysterectomy rate in the United States is higher than it should be, meaning that it may not be necessary in every case. Before you agree to the procedure, ask your doctor about alternative treatments for your condition and get a second opinion. If hysterectomy offers the best chance for your health, keep in mind that dealing with all of the physical and emotional changes that accompany the surgery can take a year or more.

Sexual Rx: The Sex Therapists' Tool Kit

Now that you're aware of the possible problems of sex, here are a few ideas for avoiding or solving them. Some of the traditional tools of sex therapy for boosting sexual response and enhancing intimacy are safe, highly effective, and fun to practice at home. They may also be used by couples whose problems are not serious enough to warrant a trip to a therapist.

Kegels

The classic sex exercise—called Kegels after Arnold Kegel, the gynecologist who developed them—are designed to improve pelvic support. They are simple contract-and-release moves that tone and strengthen the pubococcygeus (PC) muscle, which lies at the base of the pelvis, encircling the urethra, vagina, and anus.

Kegel originally developed the exercises to help incontinent women. But after treating many patients, he found that Kegels had undeniable sexual side effects. Some women reported experiencing orgasm during intercourse for the first time. Sex therapists routinely prescribe Kegels to magnify sensory awareness in the genitals and enhance sexual pleasure.

Kegels continue to intrigue researchers. In 1994, Linda Newhart Lotz, Ph.D., a sex therapist in Gainesville, Florida, showed that women who practice Kegels have more frequent, intense orgasms and a heightened ability to predict and control orgasm. Moreover, the women who did Kegels prior to sex reported that they became lubricated more quickly. That's probably because Kegels increase blood flow in the pelvic and vaginal regions.

Doing Kegels every day can help maintain strength in the vaginal muscle, improving sexual response. As with any new exercise, you can strain yourself by doing too much too soon, so it's wise to start practicing Kegels gradually. Here's how to perform them:

- First, you need to identify the PC muscle. It's the same muscle you use to stop the flow of urine. Imagine trying to stop the flow of urine midstream. This is the muscle you'll need to contract.
- You can perform Kegels anytime, whether sitting at your desk, standing in the shower, or lying down. Start by tightening the PC muscle and holding the contraction for several seconds. Gradually work up to ten seconds. The exercises will be most effective if you hold the contractions for the full ten seconds.
- Repeat the set of ten contractions several times during the day. Some experts recommend doing this as many as five times a day (fifty contractions).

Once you've mastered the basic Kegel regimen, you can try variations: Gradual Holds (gradually contracting the muscle for ten seconds, then

149

slowly reducing the tension) or Flicks (contracting the muscle quickly to a fast beat). Pumping up your PC may also help to ease menstrual cramps and strengthen the pelvic muscles weakened by childbirth.

Sensate Focus Exercises

Masters and Johnson developed sensate focus exercises as a way to enhance sensuality and arousal. Widely prescribed for people who have lagging sexual desire, they may be particularly useful to women in whom emotional and psychological issues, such as body image or communication difficulties, lurk behind the hindered sexual response.

As the name suggests, the focus is on giving and receiving pleasurable sensations. The famed sex research team realized that the overriding goal of orgasm could itself become a barrier to fulfilling sex, so the exercises involve couples exploring one another's bodies without achieving orgasm.

The program occurs in three phases. Some therapists instruct their patients to allow a certain amount of time for each stage—two weeks, for instance—before progressing to the next stage. At the end of the therapy, couples have a better understanding of their partner's unique turn-ons and pleasure points.

Therapists usually tailor specific guidance to the couple in therapy, but the basic principles can be adopted by anyone wishing to restore intimacy.

First Stage: The goal is to relearn how to give pleasure through nonsexual touch. Each partner takes turn stroking, massaging, and caressing the other partner's body everywhere but the genitals. The active partner focuses on giving pleasure, while the passive partner simply receives it.

Second Stage: The focus shifts to receiving pleasure. The exercises are essentially the same, but the passive partner communicates when touch is not pleasurable or is especially pleasurable, too light or heavy, too slow or too fast. At this phase, kissing is allowed, but the genitals are still off limits.

Third Stage: The emphasis on sensation continues, but now the partners introduce genital touch. The partners exchange turns arousing each other but stop short of orgasm. At the end of this phase the couples resume having orgasms, sharing a renewed awareness of their own and their partner's sensuality.

Directed Masturbation

When a woman is unable to experience orgasm, therapists may prescribe a technique known as directed masturbation. Women who have never had an orgasm (about 10 percent of women) can often be taught to do so. Directed masturbation is designed to help women achieve orgasm first on their own and then with their partners.

The goal is to help a women discover what is pleasurable to her and then convey this information to her partner. Studies of directed masturbation boast high success rates—usually more than 80 percent of women are able to have masturbatory orgasms at the end of therapy.

It's important to know that the majority of women do not climax through intercourse alone; as many as 75 percent of them require manual stimulation of the clitoris, as well. Although movies may suggest otherwise, not having an orgasm during intercourse is perfectly normal.

According to the American College of Obstetricians and Gynecologists, a woman using directed masturbation follows nine steps:

1. Increase her self-awareness by examining her body and genitals.
2. Explore the genitals with her fingers.
3. Identify sensitive areas that stimulate pleasurable feelings.
4. Manually stimulate those areas.
5. Increase the intensity and duration of stimulation, and use sexual fantasy to enhance psychological stimulation.
6. If an orgasm has not occurred, use a vibrator on or near the clitoris to increase stimulation.
7. Demonstrate masturbation with the partner present to illustrate what's pleasurable.
8. Guide the partner in manual stimulation, using nonverbal communication.
9. Engage in intercourse, using the "bridge" technique—stimulating the clitoris manually during intercourse.

Steps 7 to 9 can be practiced to help women who can achieve orgasm on their own but wish to have an orgasm during sex with a partner.

Jump-Starting Sex: A New Sex Therapy for Women

Sex problems are stressful. So finding ways to chill would seem the obvious first step toward a remedy. In fact, relaxation techniques are standard fare when treating low arousal and libido.

But groundbreaking research by Eileen M. Palace, Ph.D., of Tulane University in New Orleans, suggests that the opposite approach may also work. Women, she believes, may be more capable of sexual arousal if they are already in a heightened physiological state (read: rapid heartbeat and short breaths.)

Measuring blood flow in the vagina with special instruments, Palace gauged the physical responses of women with sexual problems after viewing an erotic film clip. Predictably, she found that women with a history of sexual problems were less responsive than a control group made up of women who had no sex difficulties. Palace then repeated the experiment using an unsexy "thriller"-type movie—followed by the erotic film. The result was a resounding thumbs-up: The vaginal responses of women with sexual problems increased dramatically.

Palace theorizes that edge-of-your-seat films act to jump-start the cascade of physiological processes that lead to sexual arousal. Her research, which was published in *The Journal of Consulting and Clinical Psychology,* also shows that when women are given feedback about their increased erotic state, they experience even greater sexual response. "We create a positive feedback loop," Palace says. "Those women who have positive biofeedback change their expectations and also increase their physical responses. Three minutes after the erotic film, they have the same sexual response as the sexually functional group."

In theory, other physiological triggers—such as exercise or even a dose of laughter—could also prime the pump for sexual encounters. While still a model for therapy, this new approach may prove to be a breakthrough in the treatment of female sexual disorders.

Making Love to a Man with Erectile Dysfunction

Erectile dysfunction—or impotence—affects from 10 to 30 million American men. Nearly every man has experienced erectile dysfunction at one time or another, but when a pattern develops, it can jolt a couple's sex life and both partners' self-esteem. "Erectile dysfunction is a couples' disease," says Irwin Goldstein, M.D., professor of urology at Boston University School of Medicine.

Erectile dysfunction is often associated with aging, although it is not an inevitable consequence of growing old. The problem is frequently linked with diabetes, high blood pressure, and other heart and blood vessel disorders, which reduce blood flow throughout the body and the sex organs.

A commonly overlooked source of erectile problems is the use of certain prescription drugs (*see "Pharmaceutical Sex Stoppers," page 141*). Other potential problems include surgery, prostate cancer and its therapy, spinal cord injuries, and any kind of chemotherapy. When psychological problems are implicated, therapy can help. Fortunately, such issues are often temporary.

Women whose partners have erectile dysfunction should make sure that their sexual needs are met—for themselves and their relationships. Learning new ways of intimacy may require some coaxing. Counseling can help you communicate your needs and also help you to deal with your own feelings of anger and guilt.

These options for men with erectile disorders may offer a return to some of your old patterns of lovemaking:

Vacuum Pump Device

These are plastic cylinders that fit over the penis. Air is pumped out of the cylinder, causing the penile arteries to fill with blood. The blood is then trapped by a rubber ring at the base of the penis.

Pros: Triggers a firm erection that lasts for twenty to thirty minutes with few side effects.

Cons: The vacuum device can take some getting used to, because it tends to interrupt sex. Many couples learn to incorporate the device into foreplay.

Injections

Injecting certain drugs—most commonly a drug called alprostadil—into the penis is another way to trigger an erection. The drugs start the same chain reaction that sparks a normal, spontaneous erection.

Pros: A man can inject himself ten minutes before sex; the erection lasts from thirty to sixty minutes.

Cons: Men using injections sometimes get priapism, a painful erection that lasts for several hours and requires emergency medical attention.

Pills

The newest weapon in the arsenal of treatments for erectile dysfunction, Viagra is a pill taken an hour before intercourse.

Pros: Produces a natural erection when the man is sexually stimulated. The drug has no effect when he is not aroused.

Cons: Some men get unpleasant side effects, including headaches, flushing, indigestion, and stuffy nose.

Implants

There are two types of implants: one is a flexible rod that gives the penis a permanent rigidity but is flexible enough to be tucked into his underwear, the other is a cylinder that must be extended and stiffened with fluid transferred from a reservoir under the abdominal muscle.

Pros: Implants offer men greater control and less awkwardness.

Cons: Infections can occur, requiring removal of the implants.

Future Methods

- The MUSE system (medicated urethral system for erection), recently approved by the FDA. A man squirts a premeasured dose of alprostadil in the opening at the tip of the penis to stimulate an erection.
- Erection-inducing solutions rubbed directly into the penis.

Impotence Resources

Impotence Institute of America
10400 Little Patuxent Parkway
Columbia, MD 21044
800-669-1603

Geddings Osbon Foundation
P.O. Box 1593
Augusta, GA 30903
800-433-4215
Publishes the booklet Male Impotence: A Woman's Perspective

A Word About Sexual Coercion

You can't talk about sex stoppers without mentioning forced or unwanted sex. According to *Sexual Coercion and Reproductive Health,* a 1995 report by the Population Council, sexual coercion is the act of forcing (or attempting to force) another individual through violence, threats, verbal insistence, deception, cultural expectations, or economic circumstance to engage in sexual behavior against her/his will.

One in five American women has been forced to do something sexually that she didn't want to, according to the 1994 "Sex in America" survey. At the same time, only 3 percent of men reported having forced someone to do something sexually. This disturbing discrepancy reveals that men and women are truly at odds about what sexual consent means.

Some women lack the power to control sexual situations because they are economically dependent on men. Even those who don't feel that their survival hinges on submitting to sex may still feel pressured for other reasons.

Myths about gender roles that tend to surface in adolescence contribute to sexual coercion, according to Steven Brown, Ph.D., a clinical psychologist in Highland Park, New Jersey, who works with teens. Here are a few of the persistent gender-based beliefs that help keep force in the sex picture:

- It's unacceptable for a male to be a virgin. Boys earn their manhood via sexual conquest.
- Boys are supposed to be initiators. Girls like guys who take control when it comes to sex.
- Girls want sex as much as boys, but they have to say no to maintain their reputation. Therefore, when a girl says no, she really means maybe or yes.
- If a guy is persistent and persuasive, the girl will eventually fall into his arms and be glad she did.
- Even if a girl doesn't want to have sex, it's still sex and can't really feel that bad.
- The penis has a mind of its own. Once aroused, it can't be controlled.

Girls are taught that sex is bad, so "they can't admit that they're sexual," Brown explains. "Adolescent boys say, 'The girls always say no. Eventually they come around.' That girls feel they can't say yes contributes to the problem. It's important that girls know they have a right to want sex and to enjoy it. The more we teach girls that they can say yes, the less that boys will always interpret their no's as maybe's and yes's."

Sexual coercion is obviously a societal problem. But women can help themselves feel less vulnerable by defining the conditions that make sex feel right for them. To start, women should simply ask themselves, "What does good, healthy sex mean for me?"

Envisioning good sex means defining the terms you require to go to bed with someone. "What kind of ground rules do you have about sex? Under what circumstances will you have sex with someone? What kind of setting do you want to have sex in? Many women have no answer to any of those questions," says Anne Kearney-Cooke, Ph.D., director of the Cincinnati Psychotherapy Institute. "A lot of them make decisions about sex on the spot. It's often not the healthiest decision. And it often leaves them feeling bad." Taking the time now to picture the right setup for sex is likely to help you feel more sexually empowered and better able to avoid dubious sexual situations in the future.

The capacity to develop bonds of intimacy through sex is one of the most meaningful ways to express your humanity. Roadblocks to healthy sex are not frivolous concerns. They dull the vibrancy of life by harming your general health, diminishing your feelings of self-worth, and reducing the quality of your love relationships. Educating yourself about the possible pitfalls of intimate behaviors—and arming yourself with strategies for avoiding them—are well worth the effort.

7 The Scourges of Love: Sexually Transmitted Diseases

Sex at its best enriches our intimate relationships and creates new life. But surrendering to our basic instincts may sometimes get the better of us. In the cold light of the morning after, the decisions we make in a moment of passion can come back to haunt us. Unwanted pregnancy and sexually transmitted diseases (STDs) are the cruel consequences of good feelings foolishly acted upon.

The most tragic STD is AIDS, the devastating disease that dismantles its victims' immune systems, leaving them vulnerable to life-threatening infections. Movies and television have brought home the terrible drama of AIDS-related death. And news about AIDS research and treatment has dictated health headlines for more than a decade.

As a result, AIDS has obscured the rise of other, less deadly but dangerous, sexually transmitted diseases. Twelve million new cases of STDs of all kinds are diagnosed every year, and one American in five now carries an incurable STD. STDs are more common than allergies. And many of them present harmful, long-term consequences to their victims, especially women and their unborn children.

At the end of 1996 the Institute of Medicine (IOM) released a report called *The Hidden Epidemic: Confronting Sexually Transmitted Diseases*. Among its findings were these alarming facts:

- Since 1980, eight new sexually transmitted pathogens have been recognized in the United States.
- STDs can cause serious life-threatening complications, including cancer, infertility, ectopic pregnancy, spontaneous abortion, stillbirth, low birth weight, neurologic damage, and death.
- Women and teens are disproportionately affected by STDs.
- STDs enhance the risk of acquiring HIV, the virus that causes AIDS.
- STDs account for almost 90 percent of all cases reported among the top ten most frequently reported diseases in 1995.

The STD crisis reflects our sexually schizophrenic world where underwear-clad models pout seductively from billboards while condom ads are banned. STDs, like all things connected to sex, are shrouded in shame, diverting doctors

157

and patients from talking openly about the risks and repercussions of intimate behavior.

If you are sexually active, you owe it to yourself to find out about STD risks along with smart strategies for preventing and detecting these diseases. Information, wise decisions, and a supply of condoms can go a long way toward making sex not only safe but as satisfying as nature intended.

Why STDs Strike Women Hardest

STDs afflict more women than men, and they are far more devastating in women for several reasons: Once an STD is introduced into a woman's body, her sexual anatomy—with all its internal, moist cavities—tends to promote the disease and evade detection. "There's more room to roam," says Joel R. Greenspan, M.D., M.P.H., a preventive medicine specialist at the Centers for Disease Control (CDC) in Atlanta. "Women have more at risk and have to be more responsible for STDs."

Many infections, including gonorrhea and genital herpes, are more easily transmitted from man to woman. With the possible exception of the female condom, which partially covers the vulva, contraceptives do not offer effective protection against infection. Due to their biology, women are also more likely to acquire a sexually transmitted disease from a single sexual act.

It's important to know that a woman is more likely than a man to harbor infections without symptoms, meaning a disease can quietly wreak its havoc before she even learns that she has become infected. For example, according to one recent study, as many as 85 percent of women with chlamydia have no symptoms, as compared with 40 percent of infected men. Women with gonorrhea or chlamydial infections are often not diagnosed until serious complications arise. Pelvic inflammatory disease (PID), which often leads to infertility, is one of the more serious consequences of unchecked chlamydial infections.

Once infected, women are more vulnerable to the long-term consequences of STDs. For example, human papilloma virus (HPV), which causes genital warts, increases a woman's risk for several different kinds of cancer including that of the cervix, vagina, vulva, and anus. Conversely, in men, HPV confers a greater threat for the relatively rare cancer of the penis.

Unfortunately, many women unwittingly compound their risk for long-range health woes. For instance, research has shown that women who douche frequently have a higher risk for pelvic inflammatory disease, perhaps because douching drives STD pathogens into the upper genital tract.

Risks may also increase when women fail to get regular gynecological exams or inappropriately treat bacterial infections with over-the-counter yeast cures.

STDs and Your Doctor

Health care has not caught up with the brazen new world of STDs. If you depend on your physician or other health-care providers to detect infections during routine physicals, you may put yourself at risk for serious health problems. Most doctors do not routinely screen their patients for chlamydia, the most prevalent and the fastest growing STD, despite alarming rates of infection and the fact that it often presents no symptoms. This is true for two reasons: Past tests were cumbersome to use, and doctors assumed that their patients were not at risk. "The testing technology for chlamydia has gotten simpler and less expensive over time. But we haven't gotten the word out to physicians," says Felicia Stewart, M.D., director of reproductive health for the Kaiser Family Foundation. "Patients assume they're being tested for STDs. And they're not." In fact, you may need to ask during a visit to your gynecologist to be tested for such common diseases.

According to the IOM's 1996 report, many doctors lack the training to diagnose and treat STDs, or to counsel their patients about high-risk behaviors. Many neglect to bring up sex-related issues for fear of offending their patients. In a recent Gallup poll, more than half of the respondents said that their health-care providers spend "no time at all" discussing STDs. In another study of primary-care physicians, only 31 percent asked their patients about condom use and 22 percent about their number of sexual partners. At the same time, nearly all physicians asked their patients about cigarette smoking. Data shows that people are more likely to learn about threats to their sexual health from television and magazines than from their doctors.

Moreover, many screening and treatment centers for STDs are operated through public health agencies that are geared more toward diagnosis and treatment—not prevention. Experts fear that managed care also makes disease prevention more difficult.

The Hidden Health Hazards of STDs

Most sexually transmitted diseases are not as inexorably fatal as AIDS, but they are still dangerous to you and your future children. So why aren't women informed about them?

Many STDs have no symptoms or they may mimic other conditions and, therefore, remain undetected. Almost 80 percent of female college students who tested positive for chlamydia had no symptoms, according to a study in the *American Journal of College Health.* And some of the long-term health hazards of STDs, including infertility and certain cancers, show up years after the initial infection, so they are not likely to be associated with STDs.

How common STD-related health consequences affect women:

- **Cervical cancer,** the second most common cancer worldwide, has been linked to infection with certain strains of human papilloma virus (HPV), the agent responsible for genital warts. The rate of HPV infection is steadily rising. In one study, nearly half of female college students had evidence of HPV infection. (The risk of contracting HPV can be minimized by practicing safe sex and limiting your number of sexual partners. If you contract HPV, you must get regular Pap smears to detect treatable cervical cell changes that could lead to cancer.)
- **Pelvic inflammatory disease (PID),** one of the more insidious consequences of STDs, affects one million women a year and is most often associated with gonorrhea or chlamydia. These infections initially affect the cervix, but they then spread into the upper genital tract and into the pelvis and abdominal area. PID can also cause chronic pelvic pain and discomfort during intercourse.
- PID can lead to a greater risk for **ectopic pregnancy** (the development of a fetus outside the uterus) because the infection partially blocks or scars the fallopian tubes and suspends the growing fetus. Currently about one in fifty pregnancies are ectopic pregnancies. If you have had PID, you are six to ten times more likely to develop an ectopic pregnancy as compared to women who have not had PID. Ectopic pregnancy is one of the leading causes of maternal death during pregnancy. It is also one of the most preventable causes.
- **Infertility,** another tragic result of PID, occurs when the fallopian tubes become scarred or blocked by infection. This type of infertil-

ity—called tubal factor infertility—accounts for 15 percent of all infertility in women. Almost all the cases of tubal factor infertility are the result of PID. STDs rarely cause infertility in men.

How STD-related health consequences affect pregnant women and infants:

- Pregnant women are more likely to have complications from STDs. Vaginal infections can cause inflammation in the placenta or fetal membranes and pelvic infections after vaginal delivery or delivery by Cesarean section.
- Women with STDs who are pregnant may transmit the infection to their fetus or infant through the placenta, during the birth, or as a result of breast feeding. Infections that affect fetuses and newborns include chlamydia, gonorrhea, syphilis, cytomegalovirus, genital herpes, and HIV infection. In some cases the infection only manifests itself years later.
- Infection during pregnancy can cause spontaneous abortion, stillbirth, premature rupture of the membranes, and preterm delivery.
- Babies born to mothers with certain STDs—chlamydia, genital herpes, HIV, syphilis, and gonorrhea—are prone to damage to the brain, spinal cord, eyes, and ears.
- Cytomegalovirus can lead to retarded growth, damage to the nervous system, low IQ, and deafness.
- Herpes simplex may trigger mental retardation or even death.
- Chlamydia can cause a type of pneumonia in infants.
- Hepatitis B becomes a chronic disease in as many as 90 percent of infected newborns.

A Guide to STDs

To guard yourself against infection, you must know your enemy. According to a Gallup poll conducted in 1996, one-third of adults could not name an STD other than HIV/AIDS. Less than one-fourth of Americans identified chlamydia—the most prevalent STD—in a 1997 Kaiser Family Foundation survey. "A lot of young women are at risk of having their fertility permanently damaged just because they don't know," says Felicia Stewart, M.D., director of reproductive health for the foundation.

This guide to common STDs should protect you and the ones you love. Preventing STD infections can also reduce your chances of acquiring HIV, the virus that causes AIDS.

Note: Whenever you have been prescribed antibiotics for an STD, it is important to finish all of the drug. If you don't, the STD may not be completely eradicated.

Chlamydia

The Lowdown

The fastest spreading STD in the U.S., chlamydia is a bacterial infection (*chlamydia trachomatis*) that afflicts four million women and men each year, many of whom do not know they have it.

How It Gets Around

Chlamydia can be transmitted through vaginal or anal intercourse, genital contact, and from mother to baby. Fondling, foreplay, and petting that involves contact with infected body secretions or sores can lead to what's called autoinnoculation: A woman can transmit the disease to herself by touching an infected area and then touching her eye. Chlamydia is a leading cause of blindness in developing countries, where it is transmitted from eye to eye by flies.

How You Know You Have It

Very often you don't: As many as 80 percent of women and 40 percent of men do not exhibit signs of the disease. That's why it's important to be tested for the disease if you are sexually active—even if you practice safe sex. The Centers for Disease Control recommends a chlamydia test when there is a new sex partner or when one partner engages in intercourse outside a previously monogamous relationship. But because you may not always be aware of your partners' other sexual relationships, it's smart to get an annual chlamydia test, especially if you are age twenty-five or younger. Symptoms may include discharge from the vagina, rectum, or penis; pain when urinating; cramps and lower abdominal pain in women; in men, pain in the testicles or burning and itching around the opening of the penis.

How You Get Rid of It

Chlamydia is easily treated with antibiotics. Your partner must also be treated so that you don't get reinfected. A one-dose cure is now available.

Other Things Worth Knowing

Chlamydia is responsible for as many as half of the nation's 1 million cases of pelvic inflammatory disease (PID), which often leads to infertil-

162

ity and a greater risk for ectopic pregnancy. Chlamydia facilitates the transmission of HIV. Chlamydia can cause chronic arthritis and is associated with a greater risk for premature births and complications in infants, including chlamydial pneumonia, a serious lung infection.

Gonorrhea

The Lowdown

More than a million new cases of gonorrhea (alias "the clap") are reported each year in the U.S. The disease is caused by the bacteria *Neisseria gonorrhoeae*.

How It Gets Around

Gonorrhea is spread by sexual contact—vaginal, anal, and oral sex— or it is passed from mother to baby during delivery. Gonorrhea is found in body fluids from the penis, vagina, mouth, rectum, and even the eye. If you touch an infected area and then touch yourself, you can become infected. A baby's eyes can become infected if the mother has a cervical infection during delivery.

How You Know You Have It

Sometimes there are no symptoms. More often, there is discharge from the vagina, rectum, or penis. You may experience a sore throat, difficulty swallowing, or pain with urination. Women often have lower abdominal pain or cramps, redness on the cervix, and frequent urination. Men may have pain in the testicles, swollen glands in the groin, and redness at the head of the penis. If there is an infection in the rectum, you may have blood or mucus with bowel movements.

How You Get Rid of It

Sometimes with difficulty. Gonorrhea is becoming increasingly resistant to penicillin. Some 30 percent of strains are now penicillin-resistant. Ceftriaxone is the common cure.

Other Things Worth Knowing

Like chlamydia, gonorrhea confers a higher risk for pelvic inflammatory disease, which can cause infertility and ectopic pregnancy. Open sores can facilitate the transmission of HIV. Untreated infections in the eye can cause blindness. Gonorrhea can spread to infect other parts of the body, including the joints, skin, heart, and even the brain. The results: rashes, fever, and joint pain.

Chancroid

The Lowdown

A bacterial infection caused by an organism called *Haemophilus ducrey*. There are some 3,500 new cases each year.

How It Gets Around

Chancroid is spread through intimate skin contact (direct skin-to-skin of open sores and other mucus membranes).

How You Know You Have It

You will get ragged, painful lesions on the mouth, throat, lips, anus, tongue, vagina, or penis. Sometimes the sores appear on the hands or thighs.

How You Get Rid of It

Antibiotics are the treatment of choice.

Other Things Worth Knowing

The open sores of chancroid foster the transmission of HIV. There may be a greater risk of infection from the disease from uncircumcised men. Women can carry the bacteria in the vagina with no visible sores and may unknowingly pass the infection to others.

Herpes Simplex

The Lowdown

Herpes simplex II, or genital herpes, will afflict a half million people this year. Experts estimate that 30 million people currently have herpes in an active or latent phase. Herpes simplex I, or oral herpes, refers to infections that affect the lips or mouth, causing fever blisters or cold sores. It affects 50 to 90 percent of the population. Both types of the virus reside in the nerve cells and cause periodic outbreaks. Like other viruses, herpes is not a curable disease.

How It Gets Around

Genital herpes is spread through contact with sores or infected body fluid through vaginal, anal, and oral sex. The virus, however, is shed in the absence of sores, so avoiding contact may not remove your risk of contracting the virus. Condoms do not guarantee protection because viral particles may be present on the skin around the genitals. Herpes can also be transmitted from mother to baby during childbirth.

How You Know You Have It

You will likely experience an outbreak of small painful bumps that turn into blisters and then open sores in or around the vagina or on the labia and the rectum. Men may get blisters on the penis. You may experience painful urination and irritation. The first outbreak is usually the worst; subsequent ones are less severe. The sores last about one to two weeks.

How You Get Rid of It

You can't. There is no cure for herpes, but anitviral medications can reduce the severity of symptoms, frequency of outbreaks, and the rate of asymptomatic shedding. Acyclovir is an often used drug. Famciclovir, approved by the FDA in 1995, is more powerful and only requires two daily doses. In 1998, researchers were working to develop a herpes vaccine to protect people from becoming infected in the first place.

Other Things Worth Knowing

It pays to stay healthy. Herpes has a tendency to revisit when you are stressed, running a fever, exposed to the sun, or when the body and the immune system have been otherwise weakened. Herpes outbreaks are more common during menstrual periods. The presence of herpes lesions on the cervix increases a woman's risk for developing cervical cancer. The open sores may make other infections, including HIV, more likely. Some people have fever, swollen glands, headaches, and backaches during outbreaks, especially the first outbreak. In newborns, the disease can cause severe infections that lead to mental retardation, brain damage, or death. Pregnant women with herpes are more apt to have a premature delivery or miscarriage. A Cesarean section is often recommended to limit the baby's exposure to the virus during delivery.

Syphilis

The Lowdown

Each year there are an estimated 100,000 new cases of syphilis; the disease is caused by a bacterium called *Treponema pallidum.*

How It Gets Around

Syphilis is spread though intimate contact, including vaginal, anal, and oral sex, and kissing, dry humping, petting, and foreplay. It is also passed from mother to child during gestation—it can cross the placenta—or at birth. It may be transmitted through a transfusion of infected blood.

How You Know You Have It

You can't always tell whether you have syphilis because it may reside in places where the sores cannot be seen—or they are mistaken for something else. There may be one or many sores, usually painless, on the genitals, rectum, or mouth. Even though the sores heal, the infection is not gone, so you must be treated. During the second phase of infection syphilis produces a rash on other places of the body. The rash can be flat, scaly, bumpy, round, or craterlike. Spots or sores on the palms or the soles are common. Large, moist patches can occur in the mouth or groin area. These physical lesions may be accompanied by headaches, sore throat, swollen glands, or hair loss. In the last stages of syphilis, many years later, infection can cause cardiovascular problems, brain damage, damage to other organs, and blindness.

How You Get Rid of It

Antibiotics will lay the bug to rest.

Other Things Worth Knowing

In babies, syphilis causes severe infection and other health complications, such as liver failure, pneumonia, bleeding, or damage to the brain, bones, teeth, and skin. Untreated syphilis results in death to the fetus in up to 40 percent of pregnancies. Having syphilis increases the risk of contracting HIV.

Human Papilloma Virus (HPV)

The Lowdown

HPV refers to a family of some eighty different virus strains, some of which are responsible for genital warts in and around the vagina. There are an estimated 500,000 to 1 million new cases each year. Some 40 million people in America have HPV. Members of this virus family also cause other kinds of warts elsewhere on the body.

How It Gets Around

HPV is highly infectious, and 80 percent of those infected give HPV to their partners. It is spread through sexual contact, including vaginal, anal, and oral sex. It can also be passed from mother to child during delivery.

How You Know You Have It

You may not know you have HPV because it does not always cause warts, or the warts may occur out of sight on the inside of the vagina. Visible warts can be small bumps or cauliflowerlike clusters in the genitals, anus, perineum, mouth, and throat. They can also be completely flat, white, flesh colored, brown, or pink. *Tip:* If you think you have a genital wart but aren't sure (some are on the flat side), there's an easy way to tell. Simply apply a cotton swab doused in distilled white vinegar on the suspected area for five minutes. If it turns white, HPV is probably present.

How You Get Rid of It

As with other viruses, HPV becomes a permanent resident in your body after you have been infected with it. Some strains of HPV are associated with the development of cervical cancer, but the HPV strains that cause warts are not associated with cancer. Warts may be removed, however, when they are painful or unsightly. Doctors use a variety of methods, from freezing the warts and applying acidic chemicals to lasers, heat, or conventional surgery. The method depends on the severity of the warts and whether they have recurred. Often more than one treatment is necessary, and scarring is possible. As of 1998, a vaccine for HPV is at least several years away, according to experts.

Other Things Worth Knowing

If you have HPV, you must get Pap smears regularly. This screening tool catches cervical cell changes that could lead to cancer. Certain types of HPV present a greater risk for cervical cancer than others. Don't panic if you find out you have HPV, since most types of the virus are not associated with cancer. Evidence indicates that the types of HPV responsible for external warts are not the same as those linked to cervical cancer. At present, new diagnostic techniques (such as Hybrid Capture) can help clinicians easily identify the types of HPV a woman has to gauge her risk for cervical cancer. Knowing which HPV type you have can possibly spare you from unnecessary worry and the most aggressive treatments. But you should know that a woman is often infected with more than one type of HPV.

HPV can also cause cancers of the penis and anus. Genital warts can cause problems during pregnancy. For example, a vaginal delivery may be difficult if warts are blocking the birth canal. There is some evidence that smoking, coupled with carrying HPV, further increases cervical cancer risk.

Trichomoniasis

The Lowdown

A very common vaginal infection caused by a protozoan called *trichomonas vaginalis*. No one knows how many cases occur each year because the infection is not currently reported to the Centers for Disease Control.

How It Gets Around

Trichomoniasis is spread by vaginal intercourse. It is far more common in women than in men because it does not grow well in the penis, mouth, or anus. It can be picked up from wet clothing like a bathing suit or a wet towel, but this form of transmission is rare.

How You Know You Have It

Many women experience a foul-smelling discharge that is yellow-green and frothy. Burning, itching, and redness are common, but like so many other STDs, there are sometimes no symptoms.

How You Get Rid of It

An oral medication called metronidazole clears up the infection. Your partner must also be treated, however, since he can reinfect you.

Other Things Worth Knowing

If trichomoniasis is not treated, it can cause urethritis (an inflammation of the urethra), cervicitis, or cystitis (urinary tract infection). Make sure you finish your antibiotics, and avoid alcohol when you are taking the medication.

Hepatitis B (HBV)

The Lowdown

An infection caused by the hepatitis B virus, HBV destroys the ability of the liver to process wastes. More than 1 million Americans have HBV, and more than fifty thousand people are infected each year through sex.

How It Gets Around

Hepatitis B is spread by exposure to infected blood and other body fluids. This means vaginal, anal, and oral sex are all methods of transmission. It is also spread by sharing contaminated needles and, rarely, by getting infected fluids in the eyes, mouth, or broken skin. It can pass from mother to child, either at birth or through breast milk. Five to 10 percent of infected adults and about 90 percent of babies who catch hepatitis B will carry the virus for the rest of their lives and are capable of infecting others, according to the Institute of Medicine.

How You Know You Have It

Sometimes there are no overt symptoms. Sometimes it shows up like the flu and lasts for weeks. You may experience vomiting and nausea, fatigue, loss of appetite, fever, yellow skin and eyes (the hallmarks of jaundice), dark urine, light-colored stool, or swollen glands with pain on the right side of the belly.

How You Get Rid of It

Infected persons usually get better with rest, fluids, and a good diet. You should be instructed to restrict your intake of alcohol and certain drugs. Those who have long-term complications may need interferon, a drug that helps the body fight off the virus. Hepatitis B is one of the few STDs for which you can be vaccinated.

Other Things Worth Knowing

Carriers are at risk of liver problems, such as liver cancer or cirrhosis, later in life. The risk of death is increased if the liver is extremely damaged. Some people never recover from the initial infection and suffer from "chronic hepatitis"—when the infection lasts more than six months it is considered chronic. About 10 percent of those who are newly infected become chronic sufferers.

Hepatitis C (HCV)

The Lowdown

Like hepatitis B, hepatitis C is a viral infection. More than 3 million people in the U.S. are infected, and about 150,000 contract it each year.

How It Gets Around

Needles and transfusions are major routes of entry, and you can acquire HCV through unprotected sex with someone who has acute hepatitis C or who is a carrier.

How You Know You Have It

Similar to hepatitis B, those infected with HCV may have no symptoms or may experience nausea and vomiting, tiredness, loss of appetite, yellow skin, dark urine, and abdominal pain.

How You Get Rid of It

Rest and fluids can help you recover. Some people need to be hospitalized or take drugs such as interferon.

Other Things Worth Knowing

Carriers are prone to liver problems later in life (liver cancer or cirrhosis) and may be at risk for death if the liver is extremely damaged by infection. People whose illness lasts more than six months have a chronic infection. About 85 percent of those who are newly infected become chronic sufferers.

HIV/AIDS

The Lowdown

AIDS is caused by the human immunodeficiency virus (HIV), which infects and kills the body's CD4 cells, weakening the immune system so that other infections can occur. A person who has tested HIV-positive is said to have AIDS when his CD4, or T-cell, count has dropped to a certain level or he develops AIDS-related diseases, such as PCP pneumonia, Kaposi's sarcoma, or cervical cancer.

How It Gets Around

You can contract HIV if you are exposed to HIV-infected blood or other body fluids, including semen, vaginal secretions, and breast milk. (It also occurs in extremely small amounts in saliva and tears.) How HIV is spread:

- Through vaginal, anal, and oral sex.
- By sharing contaminated needles to inject drugs.
- From mother to baby before or during the birth or through breast feeding.
- Via a transfusion with infected blood.

How You Know You Have It

Adults with HIV may feel fine for months or even years before symptoms emerge. Symptoms may include weight loss, fever, diarrhea, swollen lymph glands under the arms or in the groin, thrush (white patches in the mouth), certain cancers (including cervical cancer), and infections like pneumonia, meningitis, toxoplasmosis, and tuberculosis. The severity and seriousness of symptoms progress over a period of a few months or years. Women infected with HIV often have abnormal Pap smears or recurrent yeast infections. Indeed, chronic yeast infections are considered a marker for HIV.

How to Get Rid of It

There is as yet no cure for AIDS or a vaccine to prevent it. Doctors usually urge their patients to make lifestyle and nutritional changes to keep themselves in good health for as long as possible. Zidovudine, also known as AZT, is one of the primary drug treatments. It works by slowing the progress of the disease. In the mid-90s, a new class of drugs called protease inhibitors began to offer AIDS patients new hope. These drugs do not merely slow the disease but actually seem to halt its progress. People who take them often seem to return to a more robust state of health. But protease inhibitors are extremely expensive, can have severe side effects, and require religious use (they must be taken at regular and frequent intervals). Although these drugs hold promise in the AIDS epidemic, it is still unclear whether they will be useful over time and whether people can tolerate them for extended periods.

Other Things Worth Knowing

AIDS travels in bad company: Many doctors believe you should be tested for HIV if you have any other sexually transmitted disease, including chlamydia, genital warts (HPV), hepatitis, genital herpes (HSV)—and especially syphilis or gonorrhea. "HIV falls in the footsteps of other STDs," says the CDC's Joel R. Greenspan, M.D., M.P.H.

Can You Catch AIDS from Smooching?

In 1997 the CDC reported the first known case of HIV transmission through deep kissing. But the agency emphasized that the virus was almost certainly transmitted through blood, not saliva. The man who transmitted the virus had bleeding gums and canker sores as a result of his infection, and the woman to whom he transmitted the virus also had gum disease. The couple used condoms during intercourse but had regularly engaged in deep kissing, mostly at night after both had brushed and flossed their teeth, which can cause gums to bleed.

According to CDC AIDS expert Scott D. Holmberg, M.D., there are good reasons to rule out saliva as a medium of transmission. Research has shown that saliva contains proteins that inhibit HIV, and only minute amounts of the AIDS virus can be isolated from saliva. The CDC has always advised against deep, or soul, kissing with people who are HIV-positive and those whose status you don't know. To be on the safe side, stick to superficial (closed mouth) kisses.

Women and AIDS

Women comprise the fastest growing group of people with HIV/AIDS. Their numbers have increased from 7 percent of all patients in 1985 to 19 percent of new cases in 1995—the highest proportion yet.

But data show that women with AIDS do not get the same care as men: In a large study tracking HIV-infected men and women in thirteen different cities, women were 33 percent more likely to die than men who were comparably ill. Moreover, few women have been included in trials for new AIDS treatments, and a 1995 study suggested that females were 20 percent less likely to be prescribed AZT, one of the primary AIDS drugs. Many doctors are consequently still unaware of early indicators for HIV infection that are unique to women, such as cervical dysplasia (abnormal Pap smears) or chronic yeast infections.

It is also true that women are slower to seek help when they are sick and less inclined to speak up for their rights to drugs and treatments. Not coincidentally, some experts have noted a high rate of domestic violence in women with HIV. Battered women are often economically dependent and lack a sense of control over their lives, including—and perhaps especially—over what happens in the bedroom.

Even women who are not in violent relationships may lack the wherewithal to speak up for their health. Health-care providers may discourage their female patients from being tested for HIV—even at the woman's request—and dismiss women's real sexual health concerns.

Until medicine addresses the gender inequities in AIDS care, it is incumbent upon women to demand equal treatment.

AIDS and Pregnancy

Approximately 1,700 babies are born each year with HIV; this fact is the most distressing consequence of the epidemic. Some women do not know they are HIV-positive when they conceive, but many believe that even women who know they have AIDS have a right to procreate.

It's important to know your HIV status if you are pregnant or plan to become pregnant because there are measures you can take to protect your unborn child. Some women transmit the virus to their babies, while others don't. (Experts do not know which women will, but factors may include the amount of virus in a mother's bloodstream, CD4 levels, or the health of her immune system.) A large number of infants become infected during the birth itself.

AZT, a widely used AIDS drug, can greatly reduce the odds that HIV will be transmitted from an HIV-positive mother to her baby. According to a National Institutes of Health (NIH) study, AZT reduced by 66 percent the risk of transmitting HIV to the newborn when it was taken during pregnancy and labor. The data showed that only 8 percent of babies born to HIV-positive mothers taking AZT were infected, as compared with 26 percent of the babies born to HIV-positive women who got a placebo.

These findings have fueled a controversy among health-care providers over the issue of HIV testing among pregnant women. Some experts have called for mandatory testing of all women who are pregnant. Surveys show many doctors favor this policy because it could save money and protect the health of infants. Others believe it could lead to discrimination against mothers with AIDS. The CDC now recommends that pregnant women be encouraged to be tested voluntarily and to be made aware of the risks and treatments if they are HIV-positive. Individual states also have policies concerning how pregnant women should be counseled about HIV. Some even require testing of pregnant women or newborns. Mandatory testing for HIV, however, continues to be a hotly debated issue with serious ethical, medical, and social ramifications.

Condom Sense

The only way to protect yourself against STDs, including AIDS, is to use a condom with each act of intercourse. Research has demonstrated that consistent and correct condom use reduces transmission of many STDs. In a study of 256 European couples in which one partner was HIV-positive and the other HIV-negative, there were no transmissions among the 123 couples who used condoms regularly for almost two years. Among the 122 couples who were inconsistent in their use of condoms, however, 12 previously negative partners became infected with HIV. *(See Chapter 4, "Contraceptive Consciousness," page 49, for more information on proper condom use.)*

The Finer Points of Safe Sex

- Use a male or female latex or polyurethane condom anytime you face a possible risk. Sheepskin condoms are not recommended because they are not as impermeable as latex or polyurethane. Read the condom label; if it protects against STDs, it will say so on the package or wrapping.

- Do not use condoms past the expiration date. (Polyurethane condoms generally have a longer shelf life.)
- The female condom may offer better protection against genital herpes and genital warts than the male condom. (But if there are lesions present it's best to abstain.)
- If you can't use a condom, use of vaginal spermicides may reduce the risk of bacterial STDs, including chlamydia and gonorrhea.
- Use a dental dam or plastic wrap when performing or receiving oral sex.
- Apply a condom when using and sharing sex toys like a dildo.
- If you have any irritated or damaged tissue on the vulva (the external genitals) or in the vagina, you may have an increased risk for HIV and other STDs. Avoid intercourse until you are fully healed— and be sure to be tested for STDs.
- Avoid skin-to-skin contact during outbreaks of STDs that cause ulcers, blisters, and open sores, including cold sores.

Other ways to prevent infection, catch it early, or reduce recurrent bouts:

- Get tested—and have your partner tested—before sexual intercourse.
- Speak frankly to your doctor about your sexual history and behavior. Bring up any suspicious symptoms as soon as you notice them.
- Get Pap smears regularly, especially if you have had STDs or if you have multiple sexual partners.
- Ask to be tested for STDs before undergoing surgical procedures including abortion, hysterectomy, or insertion of an IUD. If you have an STD, you could develop serious complications afterward.
- If you are pregnant or thinking of becoming pregnant, get tested for STDs, including HIV.
- Don't douche—douching may force infectious agents into the upper genital tract, and it has no known medical benefit.
- Strengthen your immunity by exercising, getting enough sleep, and eating right. Taking vitamins A and C may boost your immune function generally.

Your Birth Control and STDs

Unless you are in a mutually monogamous relationship, you need to use a condom correctly every time you have intercourse to avoid STDs.

Instructions for Condom Use

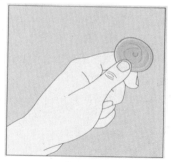

Carefully open package so condom does not tear. Do not unroll condom before putting on.

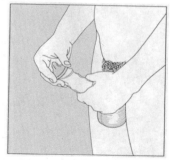

If not circumcised, pull foreskin back. Put condom on end of hard penis, leaving space at the tip.

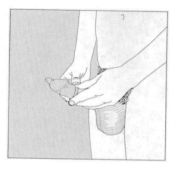

Keep rolling on condom until it reaches the base of the penis.

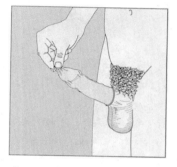

Check to make sure there is space at the tip and no breakage in the condom.

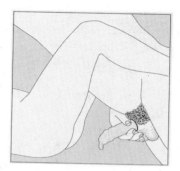

After ejaculation, hold rim of condom and pull penis out before the penis gets soft.

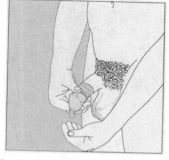

Slide condom off without spilling the liquid (semen) inside. Dispose of the used condom.

AVCS International © 1997

If you only use other kinds of birth control, you should know the following:

- Hormonal methods of contraception—the Pill, Norplant, or Depo-Provera—offer no protection from STDs.
- The diaphragm may provide some protection against cervical infection but it cannot protect you against STDs overall.
- The IUD may boost your risk for pelvic inflammatory disease (PID) and facilitate the spread of STDs from the lower to upper genital tract. It is not advised among women with multiple sexual partners or with a history of sexually transmitted diseases.
- Sterilization reduces the risk of PID from sexually transmitted pathogens, but not STD infection in the lower genital tract.

Hooked on Safe Sex

In 1988 the state of Nevada passed a law requiring brothel workers to use condoms, and for almost a decade not a single sex worker (out of more than three hundred professional prostitutes) has tested positive for HIV. By law they are also required to undergo a weekly exam for sexually transmitted diseases and a monthly blood test for HIV and syphilis.

Alexa Albert, a medical student at Harvard University, wondered how the prostitutes complied with the law and whether their safe sex strategies could be useful to other women. "It seemed like an awesome idea: If women were using condoms regularly, there might be good information," Albert says. So she spent several summers in Nevada brothels collecting evidence—literally. She inspected used condoms for holes and tears—the prostitutes achieved a zero breakage rate—and interviewed them about their habits, later publishing her data in the *American Journal of Public Health* in 1995.

The highlights of her research suggest some pointers for other women:

1. **One size does not fit all.** Prostitutes know that men come in different sizes and that condoms that are too small are much more likely to break than condoms that fit well. Professional sex workers stock up with an assortment of condom sizes. Such a strategy might never occur to many women. "They think, 'How promiscuous must it make me appear?'" says Albert. "But when do we ever buy one-size-fits-all?"

2. **Condoms go better with a lubricant.** Proper lubrication reduces friction—and the potential for condom breakage. "Having a dry vagina is the number one reason for having a condom break," Albert says. Try As-

troglide, Vagisil, or Aqua Lube—a brand favored by Nevada's sex workers because it is easy to dispense. (Avoid oil-based lubricants, which can erode latex.)

3. **Change is good.** Prostitutes stop and replace condoms during intercourse—once or even several times, especially if sex is particularly vigorous. Some sex workers change condoms as often as every five minutes.

4. **Check your mate.** Sex workers report checking the condom from time to time to make sure it is intact; others hold on to the condom's rim during the entire act of intercourse.

5. **When in doubt, double up.** That's right, two condoms are sometimes better than one.

6. **Getting it on may be easier than you think.** "Prostitutes would rarely say they have to wear a condom because it's the law. That might be perceived as unsexy," Albert says. Instead her research revealed that legal prostitutes have devised some clever one-liners to encourage the use of condoms. Here's a sampling:

"I'd make the President use one."

"I'm so hot for you, and this condom keeps you hard longer."

"I'll put it on you—with my mouth."

Whatever they're doing, it works—and their techniques may hold clues for you, too.

Interview with a Vamp

Delores French has been a professional prostitute for more than twenty years. As the founder of HIRE (Hooking Is Real Employment) and a member of the North American Task Force on Prostitution, she actively promotes prostitutes' health and legal rights.

Like many sex workers, French advocates the use of condoms, though clients sometimes resist. Even before the emergence of AIDS, French had perfected techniques for getting men to wear condoms, even sneaking them on during oral sex. Whether or not your partner knows what you are doing, French's technique offers a sensual start to safe sex:

To begin with, French favors a nonlubricated condom. "The lubricated kind tastes awful. While many experts feel that lubricated condoms are best for safety, they're no good at all if people don't use them," she says. She also likes those with no tip on the end because they can tickle the throat.

LUST IN SPACE?

Forget Tang and freeze-dried ice cream. One of the newest products of the space program is designed to give your sex life a lift. Called Astroglide, it's a water-based personal lubricant that mimics the body's natural secretions to counter vaginal dryness and increase sexual stimulation.

Astroglide was developed by a NASA chemist who discovered the extremely slippery material while working on the space shuttle and realized its potential as a medical and sexual aid—hence the space-age name. Astroglide's superlubricating properties have earned it a cult following.

Indeed, Astroglide may be the right stuff in more ways than one: Such water-based lubricants reduce the chance of condom breakage—making safe sex safer still. (For a free sample of Astroglide, call 1-800-848-5900.)

French places the condom in her mouth, tucking it into her cheek. She lubricates the penis to prepare it for the condom by licking a finger and sliding the saliva along the shaft of the penis. She then takes another finger and does the same. She repeats the task using each of her fingers, taking care to avoid putting a finger back in her mouth and potentially exposing herself to disease. "I never touch the top of the penis twice and using one finger at a time is more sensual anyway."

The challenging part is getting the condom over the head of the penis without the man's knowing it. French talks seductively, then right before she places her mouth on the penis, she moves the condom toward the front of her teeth. At the critical moment—when the condom snaps onto the head of the penis—she reaches up and pinches the man's nipple, creating a distraction. French uses her lips and tongue to slowly unroll the condom down the shaft. Making sure the condom is withdrawn properly is also key to the safety of the act, so French holds the rim of the condom at the base of the man's penis.

French also practices other safe sex activities. "Sensual cleansing" incorporates cleaning into the erotic experience. She doubles up with condoms, using plenty of lubricant to avoid condom breakage, and changes condoms frequently. "I always have plenty of condoms, and I always have several [packages] ripped open and ready," French says. "Trojans come attached [the edges are perforated]. I tear the ends off all the way along six or eight at a time and have them nearby so I can get to them very easily."

Wanted: A Topical Microbicide for Women

Becoming versed in correct (and creative) condom use remains your best protection against HIV and other STDs. But they won't protect everyone because many women lack the power to control sexual situations or to demand that men use condoms.

In the early 1990s, as public health officials begin to see that AIDS and other STDs affected women differently than men and that men were the main spreaders of disease, they identified a new research priority: a vaginal microbicide that would incapacitate viruses and bacteria in the same way that spermicides kill sperm. The female-controlled chemical method they envisioned would prevent HIV and STD transmission. The substance—foam, film, or gel—would be inserted into a woman's vagina to inactivate microbes responsible for disease and/or prevent them from attaching to the vaginal walls. According to Ward Cates, M.D., a researcher with Family Health International in Durham, North Carolina, "Theoretically, the method should be undetectable to the women whose partners might object."

One candidate is nonoxynol-9, or N-9, the active ingredient in spermicides. N-9 has been shown to destroy HIV in test tubes, though its effect on HIV acquisition during actual sex is uncertain. Studies have demonstrated that it reduces the risk of acquiring gonorrhea or chlamydia by 20 to 70 percent. But the only study to investigate its effect on AIDS transmission showed no protective benefit. Other studies were well underway in 1998. Researchers were also exploring a substance called menfegol, a spermicide that's similar to N-9.

In studying the effects of various agents on the acquisition of sexually transmitted microbes, researchers must also consider possible harm to the vagina. There is concern that N-9 can irritate the vaginal walls or disrupt the vaginal ecology, perhaps *facilitating* the spread of disease by disarming the vagina's natural protective mechanisms.

As a result, there's growing interest in kinder, gentler approaches. New classes of compounds that are less harsh include magainins and aminosterols. Magainins block the invasion of infectious organisms by punching holes in their cell walls, causing them to die. Aminosterols prevent pathogens from replicating in vaginal cells.

The Population Council, which conducts contraceptive research, has developed an experimental microbicide made of compounds known as sulfated polysaccharides. They keep HIV from attaching to the surface of the vagina and being absorbed into the vaginal mucus. Unlike N-9, an effective polysaccharide compound would allow a woman to become pregnant but protect her against disease.

Chemical barriers to STDs would offer an alternative to condoms, currently the only known way to prevent HIV and other types of sexually transmitted infections. Such compounds are not expected to reach the market before the year 2002.

The Five W's of HIV Testing

Millions of Americans are at risk for AIDS but have not been tested for HIV, the virus that causes AIDS. Half of those who are HIV-positive do not know it, according to the Centers for Disease Control (CDC). Health agencies now almost universally recommend testing to determine whether you have acquired HIV.

Who

According to the *University of California at Berkeley Wellness Letter*, you should get an HIV test if you:

- have had unprotected sex with someone you know or suspect might be infected with HIV
- ever shared needles to inject drugs
- have had a sexually transmitted disease
- had a blood transfusion between 1977 and April 1985 (before there were measures to screen blood for HIV) or have had multiple blood transfusions for any reason
- had unprotected sex with someone who might say "yes" to the above questions.

Other experts also recommend testing if you:

- have lived in an area of the world where HIV is prevalent
- have a workplace injury or accident that could expose you to HIV
- are pregnant or planning to become pregnant.

What

The test you get will probably be the ELISA. A highly sensitive screening test, ELISA does not detect AIDS itself but the antibodies to HIV-1, the most prevalent strain of the disease in the United States. (HIV-2 is a variant strain that is mostly found in people who live in West Africa.) Though it is very accurate, ELISA can sometimes register false positives, so positive results are confirmed by a second, more expensive, test, called the Western Blot.

ELISA is extremely accurate—almost 100 percent. Only one in one thousand people may have a false positive test. Almost none will test false negative.

Another less common test, the Murex SUDS test, requires smaller samples and can be processed immediately. It may also result in a false positive, making an additional test necessary. It is used in emergency rooms where quick results may be needed. Two new tests were approved in 1996: a urine test, which is not as accurate as the blood test, and an oral fluid-based test, using a treated cotton pad that collects oral fluid from between the gum and cheek.

You should receive (or request) counseling before the test and when getting the results. If you test positive, you can receive information about medications that may keep you in a good state of health for a longer period, as well as safe-sex practices to protect those you love from becoming infected.

When

To improve the accuracy of the process, have yourself tested three to six months after the last act of unprotected sex. It can take this long for your body to produce antibodies to HIV. Your best bet: Test now—and test again later.

Where

You can be tested in a doctor's office, local health department, or AIDS organization at a cost of about $100 to $200. (Public clinics offer free or low-cost tests.) For more information on where to get tested, call the CDC hotline: 800-342-AIDS.

Why

1. If you test positive, there are drugs available that can keep you healthy longer and offer better ways of monitoring the progress of the disease.

2. If you are pregnant, you can radically reduce the chances of passing HIV on to your unborn child. (Mother-to-infant transmission can be lowered by as much as two-thirds by taking AZT during pregnancy and childbirth.)

3. HIV tests are more accurate—and private—than ever. Many clinics now offer anonymous testing, and home HIV test kits are confidential.

4. You can take precautions to prevent the spread of the disease.

HIV Test Tip

If you are not tested anonymously, your tests results could make it into your medical history and possibly jeopardize your future insurance coverage. It is wise to discuss this issue before you submit to a test. Make sure that the test results—or the fact that you even got the test—will not be included in your record. If you are in the market for health insurance, wait until you are insured before you get tested.

Caution: Don't donate blood to find out your HIV status. If the infection is an early one, you may unwittingly donate HIV-positive blood, and you could pass the virus on to others. You will also be falsely reassured about your health.

Home HIV Tests

If you prefer to do your testing at home, there are several options. The FDA approved the first at-home HIV test in 1996. You can buy one at drugstores, by mail, or even via the Internet for $30 to $50.

This is how the test works: You collect a blood sample by pricking your finger and applying drops of blood to a card. You then send your specimen to the manufacturer's lab for testing. About a week later, call for your test results using a special code so that you remain anonymous.

Home-testing kits use the same technology (the ELISA—*see page 180*) for determining your HIV status as the tests at the doctor's office or clinic, but you do not have the option of getting face-to-face counseling before and after your tests, though trained personnel will talk to you by phone. In some cases, a live counselor will tell you the results if you test positive for HIV and will answer your questions. If you are HIV-negative, you may simply get a recording. Currently the only FDA-approved home test is marketed under the name Home Access (800-HIV-TEST).

Resources

National AIDS Hotline
English Service (7 days/week, 24 hours/day)
800-342-AIDS

Spanish Service
(7 days/week, 8 A.M. to 2 A.M. ET)
800-344-7432

TTY Service for the Deaf
(Monday to Friday, 8 A.M. to 2 A.M. ET)
800-243-7889

National STD Hotline
(Monday to Friday, 8 A.M. to 11 P.M. ET)
800-277-8922

National Herpes Hotline
(Monday to Friday, 9 A.M. to 7 P.M. ET)
919-361-8488

Herpes Resource Center
(Monday to Friday, 9 A.M. to 7 P.M. ET)
800-230-6039
Offers publications about herpes.

ASHA HealthLine
(7 days/week, 24 hours/day)
800-972-8500
Offers free publications about sexual health communication.

Project Inform
1965 Market Street, Suite 220
San Francisco, CA 94103
415-558-8669, 800-822-7422
Web site: http://www.projinf.org
Offers publications and fact sheets on AIDS diagnosis and treatment, a national treatment hotline, and other information.

Good Vibrations
938 Howard Street, Suite 101
San Francisco, CA 94103
415-974-8990, 800-289-8423
E-mail: goodvibe@well.com
Sells latex condoms, gloves, and dental dams by mail.

8 | Sexual Health at Midlife

Menopause—the end of menstruation and a woman's reproductive life—triggers a cascade of physiological, sexual, and psychological changes. These changes generally begin to happen to women in their forties and fifties and can linger for more than a decade, sometimes causing significant disruption.

Women experience a variety of physical symptoms as their bodies adjust to the cessation of ovulation and estrogen production. The severity and duration of these symptoms vary, depending on the woman's health, her genetic makeup, and, to some extent, her feelings about the loss of sexual and reproductive capacity.

Until recently, menopause was even more cloaked in mystery than other sexual and reproductive subjects. But thanks to the baby boom generation, which is fast entering midlife, the details of menopause have gone public. At the same time, advances in menopause-related health issues have helped to perfect the treatments and ease the myriad transitions, improving the outlook for sexual well-being over women's life spans.

Simply finding relief for menopausal symptoms often improves a woman's interest in, and attitude toward, sex. In fact, women at midlife can today expect to have healthy, satisfying sex in their forties, fifties, sixties, and beyond.

The Waning Moon: Perimenopause

Some 40 million women will go through menopause over the next two decades, but the experience will be different for each of them. The transition phase—from normal menstruation to the cessation of monthly periods—is called perimenopause, or more simply "the transition," says Donna Shoupe, M.D., professor of obstetrics and gynecology at the University of Southern California School of Medicine in Los Angeles. It usually occurs between the ages of forty-five and fifty-five, and it lasts for approximately four years. Eight out of a hundred women will start perimenopause before they turn forty, however, and five out of a hundred will have monthly periods until they are sixty.

The periomenopausal period is often marked by a number of symptoms related to the body's diminishing production of estrogen and progesterone. Egg-producing follicles in the ovaries become less responsive to the normal action of the hormone that triggers ovulation (called follicle-stimulating hormone, or FSH). This causes the pituitary gland to produce more FSH, which in turn boosts estrogen production sharply. Sometimes progesterone is not produced at all. "The ovaries are wearing out," Shoupe says. "Overall estrogen levels are falling."

These erratic hormone surges result in irregular periods and abnormal bleeding for some 70 percent of women in their forties. Other tip-offs to perimenopause: hot flashes, insomnia, vaginal dryness, and a worsening of PMS symptoms in women who have them. "Women sometimes report just feeling draggy," Shoupe says. Because the number and extent of symptoms vary from person to person, doctors sometimes fail to recognize the problem, delaying treatments that could spare women undue suffering.

Women in perimenopause may be ready for hormone therapy. Tops on the list is estrogen. "I will sometimes prescribe a low dose of estrogen," says Shoupe. Low-dose oral contraceptives can also help many transitional women through the hormone limbo, according to Valerie Montgomery Rice, M.D., a reproductive endocrinologist at the University of Kansas Medical Center in Kansas City. "There's no reason women can't stay on oral contraceptives through menopause," she says. Birth control pills and mini-pills can help regulate periods and reduce annoying symptoms while also serving as contraception.

Menopausal Symptoms

When you have had no periods for one year, you have officially reached menopause. Symptoms can become pronounced. Here are a few of the common menopausal complaints and popular remedies.

Vaginal Dryness

The loss of estrogen causes the vaginal lining to become thinner and drier, while the vagina becomes shorter and more prone to infection and irritation. The vagina produces less lubrication during sexual arousal and may do so more slowly, sometimes leading to painful intercourse. Not surprisingly, these physical problems can dull interest in sex.

Relief

Hormone replacement therapy (HRT) can be especially useful. Hormonal creams and suppositories can be placed directly inside the vagina.

Estring, a soft, flexible vaginal ring, releases a low continuous dose of estrogen for ninety days. Some practitioners may also recommend opening a vitamin E capsule and applying the oil directly to the vaginal tissue.

Many women find a quick fix to the sexual problems associated with dryness in gels and lubricants such as Astroglide and Replens. Regular sexual activity can also improve blood flow to the vagina, increasing natural lubrication. In one study, postmenopausal women who had sex more than three times a week experienced significantly less vaginal atrophy than women who had intercourse less than ten times a year. It helps to prolong foreplay and practice Kegel exercises (*see Chapter 6, "Kegels," page 149*).

Hot Flashes

Some 75 percent of women experience hot flashes/hot flushes—a sensation of sudden warmth that produces a measurable change in body temperature. The hot flash is frequently followed by a hot flush—redness, sweating, and intense heat in the upper chest, neck, face, and scalp. Some women also experience palpitations, weakness, and fatigue.

Hot flashes and flushes can persist from a few weeks to many years, usually beginning before a woman's last period. At the beginning of menopause, they may only occur at night. Nighttime hot flashes are particularly annoying because they can cause night sweats that drench nightwear and bedding or interfere with sleep, triggering irritability and depression.

Relief

Estrogen often relieves hot flashes and night sweats, but there are also pharmaceutical options if you choose not to or cannot take estrogen:

- *Clonidine.* This high blood pressure medication works against hot flashes by decreasing the production of norephinedrine, a hormone believed to regulate hot-flash signals. It can be taken orally or by patch, and side effects include drowsiness, dry mouth, and lowered blood pressure.
- *Bellergal.* This medication combines ergotamine, which causes blood vessels to contract; belladonna, a substance that helps control the body's thermostat; and the sedative Phenobarbital. Potential side effects include dry mouth and dizziness, and Phenobarbital is potentially addictive.
- *Natural and synthetic progesterone.* Though not as effective as estrogen, natural progesterone and synthetic progesterone compounds, called progestins (such as Provera), help some women control hot

flashes. They are usually taken orally. Provera is also available by injection—the dose lasts for two or three months. Some women experience headaches, weight gain, and depression. Unfortunately, the progesterone options can increase the risk for breast cancer.

Many doctors recommend vitamin E in doses of 400 to 600 international units (IU), and phytoestrogens offer an increasingly popular alternative for women who are undecided or cannot take estrogen. These natural estrogenlike substances are found in soy products like soybeans, tofu, soy milk, and miso soup. Japanese women rarely get hot flashes, and researchers suspect that their soy-rich diet may be responsible.

Edible Estrogen

When it comes to menopause, the new buzz word is phytoestrogens, hormonelike compounds that function like estrogen. Studies have shown that these chemicals, found in a variety of foods (think: soy), can provide significant symptom relief. Phytoestrogens may help explain why Japanese women, whose diet contains plenty of soy protein, don't even have a word for hot flash. In one recent study, women who ate soy-flour products reduced the frequency of hot flashes by 40 percent, while a group who consumed wheat flour products saw a reduction of 25 percent.

And there's increasing evidence that phytoestrogens—soy products and a few other plant foods—decrease the risk for heart disease and osteoporosis. Here are some foods with phytoestrogenic compounds:

Soy Products

soy milk	tofu
soy butter	tempeh
soy nuts	miso soup
soy protein	

Other Plant Foods

alfalfa	flaxseed
apples	garlic
barley	hops
carrots	peas
potatoes	rice
red beans	wheat

It also helps to pay special attention to good health measures like exercising, not smoking, and avoiding alcohol and caffeine.

Urinary Problems

The estrogen decline may also affect the urinary tract, causing the tissue to thin and reducing muscle tone. Some women experience an increase in urinary tract infections or a loss of bladder control, diminishing their quality of life. One in four women between the ages of thirty and fifty has experienced urinary leakage, according to the National Institute of Diabetes and Digestive and Kidney Disorders.

Stress incontinence results from a loss of muscular strength. Women with stress incontinence leak small amounts of urine when they laugh, cough, sneeze, or exercise. *Urge incontinence* results in a need to urinate frequently and with urgency. A woman with urge incontinence may lose urine as soon as she feels the urge. *Overflow incontinence* is the feeling that the bladder is not quite empty. Sometimes different types of incontinence occur together, says Lauri Romanzi, M.D., a urogynecologist in New York City.

Relief

Kegel exercises are usually recommended to strengthen the pelvic floor muscles. To locate these muscles, imagine stopping the flow of urine midstream. Squeeze and hold for a count of three, then relax for a count of three. Repeat squeezing and relaxing for about five minutes. Do this several times a day. You can also use weighted tamponlike cones that you hold in the vagina to strengthen the pelvic floor muscles. FemTone Vaginal Weights ($100–125) are available at drugstores without a prescription, or call (800) 422-8811 to order by mail.

Hormone replacement therapy in pill or cream form will help reverse some of the underlying conditions that contribute to discomfort and infection.

If you are still having a problem, your physician may suggest other solutions, including biofeedback to help you identify the pelvic muscles; bladder training, which can improve your ability to hold urine; certain medications that either decrease bladder contractions or help the bladder neck stay closed; balloonlike urethral plugs or patches that prevent urine leakage; collagen injections, which help strengthen the urethral sphincter muscles; or a pessary device, which is inserted into the vagina to hold the bladder neck in place.

Surgery is a last resort and is successful in 80 to 90 percent of cases. A somewhat controversial surgical technique called the laparoscopic Burch procedure involves making several dime-sized incisions instead of a traditional abdominal incision. It is less painful and has a quicker recovery time.

Other Menopausal Symptoms

- *Breast.* Some women also experience breast changes as the glandular tissue is replaced with fatty tissue, causing the breasts to sag. Nipples become smaller and flatter.
- *Skin.* The skin in general becomes less elastic and thinner. For some it becomes rougher and dry. Aging skin produces less melanin, the pigment that prevents sunburn.
- *Hair.* Hormonal changes affect the quantity and texture of hair growth. Hair may become darker, thicker, or less shiny.

In addition to HRT, which can reduce many of these changes, following good health habits—eating well, exercising, sleeping properly, and drinking lots of water—can keep you looking and feeling healthy at menopause.

Hormone Therapy: The Debate Continues

Deciding whether to replace the estrogen your body is no longer producing is not an easy decision. Hormone replacement therapy—or HRT—not only relieves the short-term symptoms of full-fledged menopause, such as hot flashes and urinary incontinence, but it also seems to counter the potentially fatal long-term health risks attributed to estrogen decline, including heart disease and osteoporosis.

Some practitioners—and patients—are wary of HRT, though, especially its possible link to cancer, which has led to heated debates in recent years. This debate is good for women. Even better: HRT has become a hot research topic. Medical scientists are churning out study after study on the long-term effects of the therapy, increasing our understanding of how these hormones affect the body.

HRT consists of estrogen combined with progestin, a synthetic version of progesterone. (Estrogen replacement therapy is simply estrogen.) The progestin is included in the therapy because it inhibits cell growth in the uterine lining, or endometrium, which can lead to endometrial cancer if left untreated. (Women who have had hysterectomies need not fear endometrial cancer since their uteruses have been removed, and they can safely take estrogen alone.)

Deciding whether to go on HRT, when to start, and how long to stay on it are complicated decisions that should be made with a physician. The discussion should include your personal risk factors, such as a family history of breast cancer. In addition, your hormone decision should be reviewed every five years or so as your needs and symptoms change, as medical researchers improve treatments, and as new data on the hormones' effects emerges. The National Institutes of Health's Women's Health Initiative has launched a fourteen-year clinical trial to identify the long-term effects of estrogen on 25,000 postmenopausal women.

Here are the important issues surrounding hormone use at present:

Heart Disease

More women die of heart disease than any other disease, including all cancers combined, and estrogen provides a strong protective benefit: It reduces total cholesterol, raising the levels of high-density lipoprotein (HDL) cholesterol—"good" cholesterol—while reducing levels of the more harmful low-density lipoprotein (LDL) cholesterol. Until age sixty-five, women are at lower risk of heart attack than men. By age sixty-five, a woman's heart attack risk is as high as a man's because of the waning estrogen levels. Studies have shown that HRT reduces women's risk of heart disease by 40 to 60 percent and stroke by about 30 percent.

Osteoporosis

HRT also seems to protect against osteoporosis, the bone-thinning disease that can cause serious bone fractures in later life. When estrogen production decreases during menopause, bone loss accelerates significantly. HRT helps to shore up this loss for as long as a woman is on it, but the greatest benefits begin during the first five to seven years following menopause. Doctors often advise women to stay on HRT for ten years to prevent or delay the onset of osteoporosis. Women with significant risk factors for the disease may be advised to take HRT for the rest of their lives. Risk factors include being Caucasian or Asian, having a small, thin frame, a family history of the disease, early menopause, lack of exercise, smoking, and childlessness.

Cancers

The data on the association between HRT and breast cancer are inconclusive so far, but some recent studies show a slightly elevated risk in women who took estrogen for more than fifteen years. Women with a family history of breast cancer may therefore be poor candidates for long-term HRT. (If your mother developed breast cancer after

190

menopause, your risk for the disease is significantly lower than for women with close family members who developed breast cancer prior to menopause.)

There is a link between estrogen therapy and endometrial cancer, especially after five years of use. The risk appears to be lessened when progestin is included in the regimen, as is the case with HRT. To further complicate matters, data show that women on estrogen who develop endometrial cancer have a higher cure rate than women not taking the hormone.

Alzheimer's Disease

HRT may reduce the risk for Alzheimer's disease, the old-age condition characterized by a progressive deterioration in brain function. In 1997, the National Institute on Aging in Bethesda, Maryland, reported that taking HRT reduced the risk of this devastating illness by half.

Method of Delivery

HRT is most commonly taken in tablet form. Pills have the advantage of increasing the level of HDL cholesterol, but if the dose is too high, it can result in unwanted side effects. Injections do not supply as steady a dose, and patches do not provide the HDL benefits of the pill form, though they can relieve menopause symptoms. Vaginal creams can be appropriate for localized symptoms like vaginal dryness.

Side Effects

Since the hormones are the same as in birth control pills, many of the side effects of HRT are similar: Estrogen triggers breast tenderness and swelling; progestin may cause water retention and mood swings. Combination therapy may result in spotty bleeding, but it usually stops over time. Taking hormone or estrogen therapy can increase your risk of developing gallstones; however, women at high risk for gallstones can safely use a patch or vaginal cream.

Only you and your health-care provider can decide what is best for you at menopause. Women with a family history of breast cancer might think twice about HRT. Having bothersome menopausal symptoms and numerous risk factors for osteoporosis would tend to strengthen the case for therapy.

It's important to know that there are alternatives to HRT for the treatment and prevention of menopausal symptoms. These include new osteoporosis drugs, such as calcitonin and alendronate sodium as well as herbs and alternative remedies. Weight-bearing exercise and adequate calcium intake play important roles in maintaining strong bones. Moreover, lifestyle changes like losing weight, exercising, and eating a low-fat diet can help keep heart disease at bay if you cannot or choose not to take estrogen at menopause.

New Hope: Designer Estrogens

Imagine estrogen compounds that would reduce a woman's unpleasant menopausal symptoms while also meeting her specific health needs, say, lowering her cholesterol or shoring up her thinning skeleton. Now imagine that these same compounds carried no risk for breast cancer.

This is the dream of scientists working in the field of selective estrogen receptor modulators (SERMs), popularly dubbed "designer estrogens." These synthetic forms of estrogen, which would offer all the benefits of estrogen without its scary risks, could make the HRT debate a fact of the past within a decade or so.

A prototype of the new class of wonder drugs is already available to women fighting breast cancer. The drug, called tamoxifen, is actually an estrogen blocker, which works by activating genes that stop the growth of breast tissue. It also builds bone density. Its downside: It stimulates uterine cell growth, thus increasing the risk for uterine cancer.

In 1998, an estrogen compound with fewer risks entered the market. Called raloxifene, the drug was approved by the FDA as an osteoporosis medication. On raloxifene, women not only built up their bone density, but also lowered their "bad," LDL cholesterol. But raloxifene does not reduce menopause-related side effects. The most recent research shows that raloxifene may reduce breast cancer risk.

Researchers in several drug companies are rapidly developing SERMs that could make the difficult choices women face at midlife a fair bit easier.

Testosterone for Your Sex Life

Move over, estrogen. There's a new player in hormone therapy: testosterone. Typically thought of as a male hormone, testosterone is responsible for sex drive in women, too. Like estrogen and progesterone, testosterone levels dip around the time of menopause, though not as dramatically as these "female" hormones.

Doctors at McGill University in Montreal have been giving the hormone in combination with estrogen to women whose menopausal symptoms include lagging libidos. While the estrogen counteracts vaginal dryness and thinning tissues, testosterone enhances the desire for sex. The FDA has approved a tablet containing both hormones, and testosterone is available on its own in patches, creams, and pellets worn under the skin.

Testosterone is not without problems, however. Possible side effects include high blood pressure, a decrease in HDL cholesterol, and a greater risk for heart disease. Some women develop excess hair, acne, or, in rare cases, liver disease. Weight gain is common. And, as is true with estrogen, not every woman with a depressed sex drive will respond to the treatment.

The Menopause Revolution: Alternative Remedies

With continuing questions about the safety of HRT, it's not surprising that many postmenopausal women—up to 80 percent—have chosen not to take it. Leave it to the baby boomers to pave the way for alternative means of treating menopausal symptoms. In recent years, many of them have dismissed their doctors' advice and sampled other means for reducing symptoms like hot flashes, vaginal dryness, and irritability. Their sheer numbers have spurred research into these unconventional remedies. While these substances are far from proven treatments, there is growing evidence to back them up.

Here are a few of the popular menopause remedies:

Herbs

- **Dang Gui (or Dong-quai).** Commonly used for PMS and other reproductive woes, Dang Gui appears to relieve hot flashes, probably by controlling the dilation of blood vessels. It may also relieve breast tenderness and insomnia. There's even some evidence that it has beneficial effects on the cardiovascular system. Taken as a tincture, extract, or powder, the herb can make you more sensitive to sunburn. It is not recommended for women using blood thinners like coumadin.
- **Black Cohosh.** This herb is popular in Germany and was used for menopausal symptoms by Native Americans. It's said to relieve hot

flashes, apparently by decreasing the amount of luteinizing hormone, which is associated with hot flashes. In one large study, 80 percent of women noticed a reduction in hot flashes, headaches, insomnia, and anxiety. The herb may also reduce fluid retention. The herb is available dried or as a liquid. It should not be taken by women with breast cancer or for more than six months at a time.

- **Chasteberry.** Purported to balance estrogen and progesterone, chasteberry may help regulate erratic periods typical during perimenopause. It's available in capsules, teas, liquid, and as dried berry.
- **Panax Ginseng.** Ginseng contains estrogenlike compounds that may help relieve hot flashes. It can also improve your cholesterol profile—raising HDL cholesterol and lowering total cholesterol. It's usually prepared as a tea. It should not be used by women with high blood pressure, blood-clotting problems, asthma, or emphysema.
- **Fennel and Anise.** Like ginseng, these herbs mimic estrogen and have mild effects on hot flashes. You can make a tea by steeping a small amount of crushed seeds.

Warning: Because herbs have not been fully researched, it's wise to use them in moderation and under the guidance of a trained herbalist. Also, the quality and purity of herbs varies significantly. If you experience any unwanted side effects, stop taking them immediately. It's essential to let your doctor know if you are taking any non-drug substances.

Other Remedies

- **Estriol.** Popular in Europe, estriol is a weak form of estrogen that many use to relieve hot flashes and other menopausal symptoms like vaginal dryness. One study found it reduced recurrent UTIs after menopause. Estriol is derived from wild yam and is sold as pills, creams, and gels.
- **Acupuncture or Acupressure.** Acupuncture, the application of hair-thin needles to specific points on the body to promote healing, has been studied for its effect on hot flashes, with favorable results. Acupressure works on the same principle. Unlike other alternative remedies, these ancient Eastern techniques cause no adverse side effects. But it's important to seek out a trained professional. The American Association of Oriental Medicine (610-266-1433) provides referrals.

The Seasoning of Sex

Sustaining sexual pleasure as we age presents new joys and challenges. Many women may find sexual expression psychologically more fulfilling because pregnancy worries and old hang-ups disappear. They're more comfortable with their bodies and more familiar with how they work.

According to the *Kinsey Institute New Report on Sex,* women become more orgasmic in their forties, as opposed to their twenties, and the orgasms are often more intense. Kinsey concluded from his research that women up to age sixty do not show an age-related decline in sexual interest. A full 90 percent of couples between ages forty-five and sixty-five are sexually active, and six out of ten women report that they are more sexually in sync with their partners, according to a 1997 survey by Wyeth Ayerst Laboratories.

Unfortunately the age advantage has a price. Women can come to feel betrayed by their bodies. Aging leads to specific physical changes—slower arousal time, a reduction in fatty tissue in the genitals, and a delay in vaginal secretions. Masters and Johnson found that women over sixty may take one to three minutes of stimulation before lubrication appears, as compared with thirty seconds in younger women.

Although hormone replacement therapy offers a solution to many of the age-related sexual changes, getting older almost certainly requires altering the patterns and rhythm of sex: taking a slower pace with foreplay, allowing time for the body to respond, and placing less emphasis on intercourse and more on other forms of sexual expression.

It's important to talk with your partner about how aging is affecting your desire for sex and your sense of your own desirability. Equally important is speaking to your health-care provider about bodily changes that adversely affect your interest in sex and your sexual response. Very often these changes can be alleviated or reversed with the proper treatment—but you will only find relief if you are assertive in seeking it.

Mental Menopause

It's not just a woman's hormones that are in chaos during menopause. The change of life can affect her emotional and psychological well-being, too. The end of fertility is often a time of tremendous ambivalence, sometimes liberating and sometimes devastating. With the work of raising families or building careers behind them, women may find the menopausal years offer the time and the perspective to launch new creative endeavors.

Negative life events often occur during this time: the death of a close relative, onset of a major disease, or the necessity of caring for an aging parent. (Indeed, the stresses of midlife can also influence symptoms; a study in *The British Journal of Psychiatry* found that life stressors were a better predictor of menopause symptoms than the actual phase a woman was in.)

At the same time, our culture tends to assign limited roles to women over fifty. Employment may be harder to find or keep, and our youth-oriented advertising industry conveys the message that women are no longer useful or valuable. While some cultures reserve special roles for women after menopause, we live in a society that seems to reject its women just when they have the most to offer.

Women themselves will prove the error in confining women to the sexist and ageist stereotypes that linger. The record shows that women are about half as likely to view menopause as a difficult, unpleasant, or disturbing event as they are to think of it positively. Women who are actually in midlife are more apt to see menopausal women as freer, calmer, and more confident. And other data suggest that as women move through menopause, their attitudes toward it tend to become more favorable. We can incorporate the many advantages of life after menopause into our inventory of healthy attitudes now, whether we're fifteen or fifty, securing happy and sexually healthy years for ourselves and those we love.

Menopause Resources

Books

Dr. Susan Love's Hormone Book, by Susan M. Love, M.D., and Karen Lindsey (Random House, 1997).

Understanding Menopause: Answers and Advice for Women in the Prime of Life, by Janine O'Leary (Penguin, 1993).

Natural Menopause: The Complete Guide to a Woman's Most Misunderstood Passage, by Susan Perry and Katherine A. O'Hanlan, M.D. (Addison-Wesley, 1992).

Menopause, Naturally: Preparing for the Second Half of Life, by Sadja Greenwood, M.D. (Volcano, 1996).

Women's Bodies, Women's Wisdom, by Christiane Northrup (Bantam Books, 1994).

The Honest Herb: A Sensible Guide to the Use of Herbs and Related Remedies,
by Varro E. Tyler (Haworth, 1993).

Publications

A Friend Indeed
P.O. Box 1710
Champlain, NY 12919
514-843-5730

Menopause News
2074 Union Street
San Francisco, CA 94123

Organizations

National Women's Health Network
514 Tenth Street, NW, Suite 400
Washington, DC 20004
202-347-1140

Older Women's League
666 Eleventh Street, NW, Suite 700
Washington, DC 20001
202-783-6686

National Black Woman's Health Project
1211 Connecticut Avenue, Suite 310
Washington DC, 20036
202-835-0117

9 | Frequently Unasked Questions About Sexual Health

Here are some answers to the most basic, pressing, embarrassing, delicate, and dangerous issues surrounding sexual health.

Basic Care and Common Concerns

What can I do about red, itching skin on the outside of my vagina?

The skin outside the vagina is a common place for dermatitis, a condition that is characterized by dryness and itching. This kind of irritation often results from tight or chafing clothing, which traps your body's heat and the moisture of normal vaginal secretions. Try keeping the area cooler and drier by wearing loose-fitting clothes.

In some women, irritation can be caused by feminine hygiene products like douches, deodorant sprays, and scented panty liners. If you suspect a product is to blame for your symptoms, stop using it and see if the problem goes away. Be sure to schedule an appointment with your health-care provider if the problem persists. Remember that douches and deodorant sprays can be harmful to your health: Douching is associated with a greater risk for pelvic inflammatory disease, and use of feminine sprays has been linked to a higher rate of ovarian cancer.

What does it mean when sex is painful?

Painful sex has many sources, including vaginal or pelvic infections, endometriosis, fibroids, ovarian cysts, vaginal dryness, vaginismus (a painful spasm of the vaginal muscles), and vulvodynia (chronic irritation of the skin outside the vagina). If sex is uncomfortable, it's important to speak to your doctor, who can identify and treat the problem that's causing the pain.

Why can't I seem to stay clean?

Many women who have an unclean feeling actually harbor an infection that a doctor should treat. Be alert to these signs of infection: unusual discharge, odor, itching, or pain. Washing regularly with soap and water is usually sufficient to keep healthy women clean.

Sometimes I notice a fishy smell after sex. Is that normal?

It's common but not normal. Women with vaginal infections, such as bacterial vaginosis or trichomoniasis, often report a foul or fishy odor—especially after sexual intercourse. That's because when semen mixes with vaginal secretions, it changes the chemistry in the vagina, making odors particularly strong. Experts agree that a fishy odor is almost always due to a condition that calls for medical treatment, so it's wise to consult your health-care provider.

Can I catch anything from a public toilet? What about the facilities at the gym?

Unless your genitalia actually touch the toilet seat, you're generally not in danger of contracting a disease in a public restroom. But to be on the safe side use seat liners if provided or line the seat with tissue. The sexually transmitted disease trichomoniasis, which is caused by a parasite, can be contracted by sitting on someone else's wet towel in a locker room or sauna. Swimming pools are safe if they are maintained according to health laws and properly chlorinated.

Sometimes I get a sudden severe pain at midcycle. Should I be worried?

No. Some women feel a pain at the time of ovulation when the ovary releases the egg. Called mittelschmerz—German for "middle pain"—it may occasionally be severe enough to be confused with a more serious condition, such as appendicitis.

I've noticed that I sometimes have heavy vaginal secretions that are especially sticky or stretchy. Is this the sign of an infection?

Changes in the consistency of vaginal secretions are perfectly normal and nothing to worry about, according to Toni Weschler, M.P.H., author of *Taking Charge of Your Fertility: The Definitive Guide to Natural Birth Control and Pregnancy Achievement.* Just prior to ovulation, estrogen causes the cervical mucus to become more elastic, which makes it easier for sperm to travel through the reproductive tract and fertilize an egg. The mucus produced at this time is often compared to raw egg whites. After ovulation has occurred, production of the hormone progesterone increases, altering the mucus again and slowing sperm movement. Normal vaginal secretions are clear and white through the entire cycle.

Is something wrong if my cycle is only twenty-three days long?

No. Although the average menstrual cycle is twenty-eight days long, some women have cycles as short as twenty-one or as long as thirty-eight days. A twenty-three-day cycle is perfectly normal.

Ever since I started taking Prozac, my love life has suffered. What can I do?

The newer antidepressants like Prozac or Zoloft—called serotonin reuptake inhibitors (SSRIs)—often produce sexual side effects, from loss of desire to insufficient lubrication. Now doctors are experimenting with weekend "drug holidays." In studies, Anthony Rothschild, M.D., a psychiatrist at the Harvard Medical School, found that patients on Paxil and Zoloft enjoyed a respite from their sexual symptoms when they took a three-day break from their drugs, and the patients' moods stayed stable. (Unfortunately, the strategy did not work for Prozac, which takes longer to leave the body.) If you think your sexual problems are due to a drug, talk to your doctor about switching to another antidepressant. Another option: St. John's wort, an herbal antidepressant popular in Germany that appears to have no sexual side effects.

I have constant burning and pain on the skin outside my vagina. What can I do?

The first course of action is to identify the problem with the help of a doctor. Your condition may be vulvodynia, a little understood disorder characterized by burning, rawness, stinging, or irritation to the vulva and vaginal opening. There are many causes for the problem, including inflammation of the nerves, abnormal vaginal discharge, low estrogen levels, or a high concentration of a chemical called oxalate in the urine. Some possible remedies include antidepressants (especially if a nerve disorder is suspected), a low-oxalate diet, cortisone ointments, and biofeedback. For more information, call the National Vulvodynia Association, 301-299-0775.

Is it possible to lose a tampon in my vagina?

Absolutely not. Except for the minuscule hole in the cervix that leads to the uterus, the vagina is virtually a dead end.

Every time I get intimate with my partner, my muscles get tight, and intercourse is impossible. What's wrong?

It is possible that you are suffering from vaginismus, a painful spasm of the vaginal muscles stemming from a psychological or medical problem. Vaginismus makes sex (or the insertion of a speculum or tampon) impossible. Discussing the problem with a physician can help identify the source of the difficulty and find a solution. Counseling coupled with a gradual dilation of the vaginal opening is the usual course of treatment.

I've been diagnosed with an ovarian cyst. Does that mean I can get cancer?

Not usually. An ovarian cyst is simply a fluid-filled sac that forms on the ovary during the normal processes of ovulation. They are not linked to an increased risk for cancer. But they can be a nuisance. Cysts may cause pain and irregular periods as well as painful sex. Most cysts disappear on their own after a few months, but if they don't—or if they are large—the doctor may prescribe birth control pills, which may help shrink the cyst. Surgery may be called for when cysts are very large or are causing severe pain.

My health-care provider suggested I examine my external genitals each month along with the breast self-exam. Is this new?

Most health-care providers are recognizing the value of the vulvar self-exam. According to R. Allen Lawhead, M.D., chairman of the Department of Obstetrics and Gynecology at Georgia Baptist Medical Center in Atlanta, it is a simple, inexpensive way to safeguard your reproductive health. Women who perform it regularly can detect common skin disorders as well as vulvar cancer, a rare but deadly cancer. Here's how to do it: Sit down on a soft surface such as a bed or chair or carpet in a well-lit area. Hold a mirror in one hand and use the other to expose the tissue of the vulva (the external genitals). Look for any change or new growth, including new moles, warts or other growths; changes in skin color, especially white, red, or darkened areas; sores and ulcers (unless they were caused by an injury); and areas that are inflamed, irritated, or itching. Report any changes to your health-care provider.

I'm scheduled for a hysterectomy. What will sex be like afterward?

Hysterectomy, the removal of the uterus, can change sex in several ways. The good news is that hysterectomy should not change your capacity to have an orgasm, since sensation and arousal happen in the vagina and clitoris. After the procedure, however, women cease to have uterine contractions during orgasm, which can affect their sexual experience. Also, hysterectomy typically shortens the vagina. (Trying different sexual positions—particularly the woman-on-top position—can help alleviate any discomfort during intercourse.) In some cases, doctors may be able to perform so-called cervix-sparing surgery, which may have less of an impact on sexual functioning. "Studies support the fact that if the cervix is left in place, women don't report a change in sexual response," says Beverly Whipple, Ph.D., an associate professor of nursing at Rutgers University in Newark, New Jersey, and president of the American Society of Sex Education Counselors and Therapists.

If the hysterectomy involves the removal of the ovaries, it produces changes that affect a woman's body in a similar way to menopause. Some women report lowered libido, lack of lubrication and dry, thinning tissue, but hormone replacement therapy can usually ease these symptoms. Over-the-counter lubricants provide a quick fix.

I had an ovary removed because of a cyst. Can I conceive with just one ovary?

Your chances of conceiving are the same as before you had an ovary removed because your remaining ovary resumes the functions of the other. It will produce the hormones estrogen and progesterone and release a egg every month on schedule.

Do I have to have an orgasm to conceive?

No. Although a woman's orgasm seems to move the sperm into the upper reproductive tract more quickly, it is not necessary for conception. Conception occurs when an egg is released from one of a woman's ovaries and travels into the accompanying fallopian tube. Semen released during ejaculation contains millions of sperm that race through the uterus and into the fallopian tubes. Fertilization occurs when a single sperm penetrates the waiting egg. The fertilized egg then travels from the fallopian tubes into the uterus, implants inside the uterine wall, and eventually grows into a fetus.

The cream I bought to stop the itching "down there" doesn't work. Why not?

Many women believe that any vaginal infection must be a yeast infection and reach for a nonprescription yeast remedy to treat themselves. But the problem could be something else altogether. Other common vaginal infections, such as bacterial vaginosis and trichomoniasis, also cause itching but these problems require an antibiotic.

Only your health-care provider can say for sure what your problem is. Using a yeast treatment inappropriately can mask another infection, making diagnosis more difficult and delaying treatment. Experts say only women who have recurrent yeast infections and are sure they can recognize the symptoms are the best candidates for nonprescription yeast remedies.

What am I doing wrong that causes yeast infections?

It's unlikely that you are causing your yeast infection. Many things can disturb the vaginal ecology causing an overgrowth of naturally occurring organisms like yeast. For example, some women get yeast infections after they go on the Pill because the hormones alter their vaginal environment. Taking a course of antibiotics can also trigger a yeast imbalance by killing off "friendly" bacteria along with the unhealthy ones.

Can eating or douching with yogurt help?

Here's a practice that the experts don't agree on. Some doctors believe that eating yogurt or placing it in the vagina will help maintain the balance of microorganisms that keep it free from infection. In fact, a recent study by Israeli researchers showed that yogurt containing *lactobacillus acidophilus* reduced the incidence of both yeast infections and bacterial vaginosis when consumed regularly.

But according to Sharon Hillier, Ph.D., the active cultures in yogurt are not in the same "family" as those that naturally inhabit the vagina. Her research suggests that yogurt is unable to recolonize the vagina. The bottom line: Eating yogurt with live, active cultures cannot harm you, and if you are a woman of childbearing age, the calcium could be good for your bones.

Can I wear a tampon overnight, or does that increase my risk for toxic shock syndrome?

In 1993 the Food and Drug Administration revised its guidelines about tampon use. According to the agency, the length of wear is not associated with an increased risk of toxic shock syndrome (TSS), which is caused by a harmful bacteria. The new guidelines increase the length of time tampons can be safely worn from six to eight hours, so overnight use is okay. If you wear tampons for any length of time, you run a slight risk of developing TSS, so be alert to the disease's symptoms: a high fever, nausea, a red rash, rapidly falling blood pressure, diarrhea, muscle aches, and flaking skin.

I don't feel fresh unless I douche. Is that normal?

It depends. If you are douching to cover up an odor or get rid of a discharge, you may have an infection that a doctor should treat. You may not be aware that the healthy vagina has a "self-cleaning" mechanism due to the activity of tiny organisms called lactobacilli, which manufacture a continuous supply of hydrogen peroxide. You should also know that douching has no medical benefits; in fact it has been linked to a greater risk for pelvic inflammatory disease.

What's the best way to stay clean and fresh "down there?"

If you are in a general state of good health, you probably need to do no more than bathe or shower regularly with soap and water.

Is it safe to use tampons when I'm not menstruating to stop vaginal discharge?

It's not a good idea to use tampons for normal vaginal secretions. Using a tampon when there is little moisture to absorb can dry out the vaginal environment, making it more receptive to infections.

Where is my G-spot?

The G-spot is located on the upper front wall of the vagina, which may be difficult to reach with your finger. Try sitting on a toilet seat or the edge of a chair and exploring the front wall while applying downward pressure from the abdomen, suggests Beverly Whipple, Ph.D., associate professor of nursing at Rutgers University and president of the American Society of Sex Educators, Counselors and Therapists. You'll know you've found it when you feel a slight swelling between your fingers.

Gynecological Visits/Pap Smears

I've noticed an unusual discharge, odor, and itching. Will the Pap smear pick up any infection I might have?

The Pap smear is a screening tool for cervical cancer. It was designed to pick up cellular changes in the cervix—not vaginal infections. So don't assume that infections will be caught as a matter of course during your routine visit. If you are having symptoms like odor, itching, and discharge, it's wise to tell your physician about them. In a recent Gallup poll, nearly 50 percent of doctors reported that they did not treat the most common infection, bacterial vaginosis, if patients didn't complain of symptoms—even when doctors noticed that it was present.

THE MOST COMMON VAGINAL INFECTIONS	
Infection	Main Complaints
Bacterial Vaginosis	Thin, milky-white or gray discharge, fishy odor, itching
Yeast Infections	Odorless cottage cheese–like discharge, itching and burning
Trichomoniasis	Yellow or green frothy discharge, foul or fishy odor, sometimes itching and painful urination

How can I tell if I have an infection that a doctor should look at?

The three most common vaginal infections have a way of making their presence known. If any of these symptoms occur, it's time to get checked out.

How often do I need to get a Pap smear?

The American College of Obstetricians and Gynecologists recommends all women who are sexually active or over the age of eighteen undergo a yearly Pap test and pelvic exam. After three consecutive satisfactory smears with normal findings, the Pap test may be performed less frequently at your doctor's discretion. (Women with one or more risk factors—multiple sexual partners, smoking, history of STDs, and onset of sexual activity before age twenty—may be advised to get a Pap smear once a year.)

The most embarrassing part of my gynecological visit is the rectal exam. Is it really necessary?

The rectal exam should be an essential part of your pelvic exam. It allows your doctor or other health-care provider to gain access to areas behind the vagina and can be helpful in identifying several health conditions such as ovarian cysts or tumors, endometriosis, certain infections, and abnormal growths in the colon. The provider may also take this opportunity to screen for blood in the stool. This portion of the exam is probably when you feel most vulnerable, but it only lasts a few seconds.

Does an abnormal Pap smear mean I have cancer?

The great majority of abnormal Pap smears do not indicate the presence of cancer. For example, an abnormal Pap smear can hint at a variety of conditions, including bacterial or yeast infections, which can be treated easily. (Your doctor may then perform a more accurate test to detect these problems.) Many times abnormal lesions simply disappear on their own without treatment, so you may be advised to return at a later date for a follow-up Pap smear—say, in three or six months—to see if there has been change. If the results of your initial smear appear more serious, the doctor may remove some of the tissue for a closer inspection.

My Pap smear was "unsatisfactory." What does that mean?

An unsatisfactory result means that your sample was simply inadequate—either there were not enough cells to make a meaningful evaluation or the cells were taken from the wrong area of the cervix. You need to be retested.

What does precancerous mean? And what is the treatment?

It's important to know that precancerous cells (also called dysplasia) may or may not develop into cancer. Dysplasia occurs when cervical cells change and begin to look like cancer cells. The difference is that precancerous cells have not invaded nearby healthy cells. They have the potential to become cancerous, however, and should be treated promptly.

When precancerous cells are found, your Pap smear result will be categorized as being either low-grade squamous intraepithelial lesions (LGSIL) or high-grade squamous intraepithelial lesions (HGSIL). If a Pap smear suggests that cells are mildly precancerous (LGSIL), the doctor may do nothing and repeat the test in several months. If the dysplasia is moderate or severe (HGSIL), doctors will examine the cervix more closely and possibly remove the precancerous tissue.

FYI: Only about 20 percent of cases in which smears indicated the presence of precancerous cells develop into cancer.

My friend told me that smoking causes cervical cancer. Is that true?

Women who smoke are four times more likely to develop cervical cancer than women who don't. It is only one of several factors that can increase your risk of developing cervical cancer. Here are some others:

- Having three or more sexual partners over a lifetime.
- Beginning sexual relations before the age of twenty.
- A history of sexually transmitted diseases or viral infections such as human papilloma virus (HPV).

THE PAP SMEAR

What It Does Well
- Show cancer cells or precancerous cell changes.

What It Doesn't Do So Well
- Pick up the presence of yeast and bacteria that may indicate infection (because the Pap smear is not a sensitive test for common vaginal infections, doctors do not rely on it for this purpose).
- Show cell changes that are consistent with HPV.
- Identify changes that indicate the presence of chlamydia or herpes (but these infections may be present even when the Pap smear does not reveal such changes, so other tests may be necessary to detect these STDs).

What It Does Not Do
- Detect ovarian cancer or cancer of the uterus.
- Diagnose a woman for HIV, the virus that causes AIDS.
- Reveal endometriosis.

If I get a normal Pap smear, does that mean I don't have ovarian cancer?

No, the Pap smear cannot tell you or your doctor whether or not you have ovarian cancer. Its primary job is to detect cellular changes in the cervix that may indicate the presence of *cervical* cancer. But the Pap smear gives doctors clues about several other health problems.

How important are the new Pap test technologies I keep reading about?

Three new advances promise to improve the accuracy of Pap smear readings. Request these technologies if you are at increased risk for cervical cancer or just want a little extra reassurance. But keep in mind the most important safeguard against cervical cancer is simply getting the Pap test on schedule.

- The *Autopap 300 System* makes it possible for labs to double-check Pap smears, using imaging technologies. The system picks out the most suspicious-looking smears for a second look by a cytologist.

- The *Papnet System* also rescreens Pap smears that a cytologist has found to be normal. It selects the most worrisome cells from each smear and enlarges them on a large color video monitor for further evaluation.

• The *Thin Prep 2000 System* reduces the number of samples judged unreadable because of blood or mucus. The instrument used to collect cells from the cervix is rinsed in a vial with a preservative, then sent to a lab where the cells are filtered out and tested.

Contraception

What do I do if I forget to take birth control pills two days in a row?

If you miss two pills in a row, take two tablets as soon as you remember them and two the next day. Then resume your normal schedule. To be on the safe side, use a backup method of birth control for seven days after you first missed the pills.

If I get sterilized, does that mean I will go into menopause?

No, because sterilization does not affect the ovaries, which produce the hormones necessary for menstruation. Tubal ligation, the most common form of sterilization in women, involves cutting and tying off or cauterizing the fallopian tubes so as to prevent the egg from traveling to the uterus. Other reproductive functions continue as they did before the procedure.

On weekends I sometimes forget to take my Pills. How can I remember?

Taking the Pill on schedule is key to its superb effectiveness, so it's important to find strategies that will keep you on track. Try to associate pill taking with something you do every day—preferably at the same time of day—such as brushing your teeth. And keep the pills in sight—on a vanity or shelf—not in a drawer.

My partner's condom keeps slipping during sex. Is there anything I can do to keep it in place?

Yes, using a lubricant can help. Studies have shown that the use of additional lubricant also decreases the risk of the condom breaking, improving its effectiveness. Just make sure to use a water-soluble product. Oil-based lubricants can erode the latex in condoms.

After my partner and I made love last night, I realized I never put in my diaphragm. Is there anything I can do to make sure I don't get pregnant?

For starters, try not to panic. Fortunately there is a solution: emergency contraception. It refers to three methods of birth control that can be used after unprotected intercourse to prevent pregnancy: oral contraceptives, mini-pills, and the copper IUD. You can ask your doctor about these methods, or call the Emergency Contraception Hotline (800-584-9911), which outlines the options and will put you in touch with local providers who can prescribe them. Experts say wider use of emergency contraception could reduce the number of unintended pregnancies in the United States by 1.7 million each year.

How often should I get my diaphragm refitted?

You should have your diaphragm refitted once every eighteen months, if you gain or lose more than ten pounds, and after pregnancy. You may also want to consider having it refitted if you experience discomfort or recurring urinary tract infections.

I'm curious about the female condom, but I'm worried that it's not as good as a regular condom. What's the difference?

To start with, the female condom, which is marketed under the brand name Reality, is made of polyurethane. Most male condoms are made of latex. Reality has two rings—one holds the condom in place inside the vagina, the other stays outside and partially covers the external genitals. Reality is slightly less effective than the male condom in preventing pregnancy, but it has some advantages:

- It can be inserted up to eight hours before intercourse.
- It may be more protective against some sexually transmitted diseases than the male condom because it covers the skin around the opening of the vagina.
- People who are allergic to latex can use Reality safely without fear of a reaction.

Are IUDs safe?

IUDs are extremely safe and effective for women who are not at risk for sexually transmitted diseases. Women who use IUDs have an increased risk for pelvic inflammatory disease, so if you have ever had an STD, you are not a good candidate for the device. Because of the enhanced risk of pelvic infections, which can affect fertility, the IUD is most often prescribed to women who have completed their childbearing. Although a fish-shaped IUD called the Dalkon Shield caused miscarriages and deaths among women in the 1970s and 1980s, the types of IUDs that are currently available are safe and effective. According to James Trussell, Ph.D., director of population research at Princeton University, the IUD is highly underused.

I heard about a birth control implant that you wear under the skin for several years. How does it work?

You're probably thinking of Norplant, six silicone capsules that are placed under the skin in the upper arm. The capsules release synthetic progesterone for five years and offer excellent contraceptive protection. If you are certain you don't want to get pregnant for a good while, Norplant may be right for you. It may also be a good option if you have completed childbearing but are not ready to take the permanent step of sterilization.

If you decide to try Norplant, you may experience some side effects, including irregular bleeding and headaches. Occasionally, users have had trouble with removal, including pain and scarring. Keep in mind that Norplant offers no protection whatsoever against STDs.

I want to go on the Pill, but I'm concerned about gaining weight. Is it inevitable?

No. It turns out you are just as likely to *lose* weight as you are to gain it after starting oral contraceptives, due to the effects of the hormones on your body. If you do experience weight gain as a result of birth control pills, your doctor may be able to switch you to a different formulation that doesn't influence your weight. Those women who do put on weight from the Pill rarely gain more than ten pounds.

When I stop taking the Pill, can I get pregnant immediately?

It is likely that you will experience some delay in getting pregnant—two to three months on average—after going off the Pill. In a small percentage of women, the menstrual cycle may be delayed for several months. It's best to wait at least three months before trying to conceive.

If I get pregnant while I'm on the Pill, can it hurt the baby?

If you become pregnant while on the Pill, it is not likely to hurt the baby because the hormone levels are so low. Research does not show a significant increase in birth defects due to the effects of the Pill.

I like the idea of taking a pill every day and not having to worry about getting pregnant. But can't the hormones hurt me over time?

Many experts believe that today's low-dose Pill has many benefits and far fewer risks than the original Pill, which was introduced in the 1960s and later linked to heart disease and stroke. Most of the health problems associated with the first oral contraceptives were related to their high hormone levels. Today's pills generally have one-tenth the progestin and one-fourth the estrogen as the earlier versions.

Current research shows that the Pill actually protects women against endometrial and ovarian cancers as well as reducing the risk of benign breast lumps, ovarian cysts, and pelvic inflammatory disease (PID). It does not appear to increase the risk for breast cancer long-term. But the Pill is not for everyone. It is especially ill-advised for women who smoke.

My husband and I have all the children we want and don't want to worry about birth control anymore. Which one of us should get sterilized?

Both vasectomy and tubal sterilization are nearly 100 percent effective in preventing pregnancy. Vasectomy is the preferred method of sterilization if you look at the choice just in terms of cost, convenience, and safety. The decision is different for every couple, however, and also depends on psychological factors.

Ever since going on the Pill, I've noticed some brown patches on my face, like suntan. What is it?

What you're experiencing is a harmless darkening of the skin pigment, called chloasma, or the "mask of pregnancy." As the name implies, this darkening of the skin sometimes happens to women who are pregnant. Because taking the Pill "mimics" pregnancy by halting ovulation, this side effect can also pop up in women on oral contraceptives. The most common areas of chloasma are the upper lip, forehead, and under the eyes. The darkening usually disappears after a woman goes off birth control pills, but in a few cases it can be permanent.

I like the effectiveness of the IUD, but it goes against my religious beliefs. Doesn't it work by preventing a fertilized egg from implanting in the uterus?

That's what the experts used to think. In fact, the IUD, or intrauterine device, apparently prevents fertilization by inactivating either the egg or the sperm. How is not exactly known, but IUDs do not appear to work by preventing the implantation of a fertilized egg. Some studies suggest that IUDs may work by immobilizing sperm or by speeding the egg through the fallopian tube before it can become fertilized.

Sexually Transmitted Diseases

How can I avoid getting herpes from my husband?

The best way to avoid becoming infected is to use a condom and to avoid sex when your partner has blisters—the painful sores or ulcers that accompany herpes infection. But it is still possible to get herpes from an infected sexual partner even when there are no sores. Wearing a condom

211

provides some protection from this viral "shedding." And the female condom may be somewhat more protective than male condoms against viral shedding because it covers more territory.

Taking an antiviral medication, such as acyclovir, can reduce the frequency and severity of outbreaks—and the rate of shedding when there are no blisters.

I was treated recently for an infection, but the symptoms have returned. What's up?

One of two things could be the problem. First, it's important to take any antibiotic you are prescribed as directed. Often alcohol can interfere with its effects. You should always finish the prescription even if your symptoms have subsided. Second, if you were treated for a sexually transmitted bacterial infection, such as chlamydia or gonorrhea, but your partner was not, it's possible that your partner still has the bacteria and has reinfected you. If your doctor gives you a prescription for an antibiotic, it's important to ask whether your partner should also be treated.

My doctor told me I have genital warts. What are my chances of getting cervical cancer?

Genital warts—painless flat or raised, pink, white, or brown growths—are caused by human papilloma virus (HPV), which refers to some eighty different virus strains. Certain strains of HPV have been associated with an increased risk for cervical cancer, but these are not the same types that cause genital warts. You may still wish to have the growths removed if they are uncomfortable or embarrassing to you. Your health-care provider can freeze them, apply topical drugs, or remove them with lasers or regular surgery. The warts may recur, however.

Even though genital warts are caused by strains of HPV that are not associated with cervical cancer, it is still important to get regular Pap smears. You should also be aware that you may be infected with more than one strain of HPV.

I heard about an infection that can cause infertility without causing symptoms. Should I ask my doctor to be tested?

You may be thinking of chlamydia or gonorrhea, two sexually transmitted diseases (STDs) that may not trigger any symptoms but can have long-term health consequences. The most serious risk is pelvic inflammatory disease (PID), which happens when infections spread from the cervix to the uterus, fallopian tubes, and ovaries, sometimes leading to infertility and ectopic pregnancies. Women who are sexually active should probably ask to be tested for these STDs. Even if you are in a stable, monogamous relationship, you may want to be tested just once, according to Linda Alexander, president of the American Social Health Association. (For more information, call the National STD Hotline, 800-227-8922.)

I have herpes and want to get pregnant. What can I do to keep the baby from getting it?

The first step is to make sure your doctor knows that you have herpes. You will be closely observed at the beginning of labor to determine whether you are having an active outbreak, which could be harmful to the baby. If you have an outbreak, you may be advised to have a Cesarean delivery because the baby can become infected during a vaginal delivery. Herpes infections can cause eye problems, brain damage, and even death in a newborn. If the herpes is dormant at the time of delivery, a vaginal delivery is not dangerous.

Women who have their first herpes outbreak while pregnant are more likely to pass the virus on to their baby, so it's wise to notify your doctor immediately if you notice the symptoms of herpes: itching or burning in the genital area, sores, and often a mild fever.

Can I be vaccinated against herpes?

At present there is no vaccination for herpes, but there could be one in the near future. Several companies are conducting trials of promising vaccines.

Can you catch AIDS from kissing?

Although HIV is found in saliva (in low concentrations), there are no known cases of AIDS being transmitted through just kissing, and researchers recently found a clue to help explain why. Saliva contains a chemical that has been shown to block HIV from infecting cells. Called secretary leukocyte protease inhibitor, or SLPI, the chemical attaches to the surface of blood cells and appears to repel the virus.

I've heard monogamous, heterosexual women are not at risk for AIDS. Is this true?

Not completely. To avoid any risk of contracting AIDS, the partners must be mutually monogamous. That means neither partner is having sex with anyone else. To be protected from infection with HIV, both partners must have had sex with no one else during the last six months, *and* each partner must have tested negative for HIV. Moreover, both partners must not have injected illegal drugs or shared needles during the last six months.

Why should I be tested for AIDS?

Learning your HIV status is important for several reasons. The newest drugs for treating AIDS can keep you healthy longer, but they seem to work best if you begin taking them before you show signs of illness. Moreover, women who become pregnant can reduce the chances of passing HIV on to their unborn children by taking AZT, an AIDS drug.

Why can't I find out about my HIV status by donating blood?

Donating blood as a way to test for HIV is a risky proposition as well as being morally irresponsible. If the infection is in an early stage, donors may not test positive but can still donate infectious blood, potentially endangering those who receive it. The donor may also be falsely reassured about their own health.

How accurate are home HIV test kits?

Home-testing kits use the same technology as the tests available at doctors' offices and clinics and are extremely accurate. They are available in drugstores, by mail, or even via the Internet for about $30 to $50.

How can I get my boyfriend to use a condom?

Remind your partner that wearing a condom protects both of you from getting infections that you may not know you have, and it's possible to transmit infections even if you have unprotected sex only once. If he objects to condoms on the grounds that they are unsexy, suggest ways to incorporate them into the act of lovemaking. Unless you have both been tested for HIV, and neither of you has had unprotected sex in the last six months, wearing a condom is the only sure way to be protected from HIV and other sexually transmitted infections.

Urinary Problems

Why does sex cause urinary tract infections in some women but not in others?

Most urinary tract infections, or UTIs, are caused by a bacteria called E. coli, which normally lives in the lower intestine. Sexual intercourse provides a good opportunity for bacteria to find its way into the wrong place—your urethra. From there it's just a short trip to the bladder, where the bug flourishes, triggering symptoms. That's why women who are suddenly having sex more frequently (newlyweds, for instance) may find themselves with a UTI. Some women may have a genetic predisposition to urinary tract infections or weaker immune systems.

How can I avoid urinary tract infections?

UTIs are very often associated with sexual intercourse, but love doesn't have to hurt, according to Tamara Bavendam, M.D., director of the Center for Pelvic Floor Disorders at Allegheny University of the Health Sciences in Philadelphia:

- Clean yourself before and after sex to keep the genital area clear of harmful bacteria.
- It's important to urinate immediately after sex to prevent bacteria from adhering to bladder walls.
- The day after sex, make it a point to drink plenty of water and urinate frequently to keep the bladder flushed.
- In general, drink plenty of fluid, and try to urinate every three or four hours.
- If a couple has anal intercourse, it's important for the man to thoroughly clean his penis before entering the vagina.

Could my diaphragm be causing my recurrent bladder infections?

Yes, the use of diaphragms has been linked to an increased risk of cystitis. A recent study from the University of Washington at Seattle followed eight hundred sexually active women for six months. The women who used a diaphragm with a spermicide were more likely to develop cystitis, probably because the spermicide alters the vaginal environment, allowing cystitis-causing bacteria to flourish. A possible alternative: the cervical cap, which fits more snugly over the cervix, preventing the spermicide from leaking and disrupting the vaginal ecosystem.

Are there any drugs that relieve the symptoms of cystitis?

Yes, there are several now available. Methenamine (Prosed, Urised) relaxes the bladder muscles, reducing the need to urinate. Phenazopyridine hydrochloride (Pyridium) is an analgesic that is often prescribed to ease the burning and pain. Lower-strength nonprescription versions of phenazopyridine hydrochloride (Prodium, Uristat) are also available. Be aware that phenazopyridine hydrochloride can turn your urine bright red, and methenamine will make it blue.

Is cranberry juice really good for urinary tract infections?

Turns out this folk remedy for preventing UTIs has more than a kernel of truth. Researchers at the Harvard Medical School found that drinking cranberry-based beverages daily helped ward off UTIs. The reason: Cranberries contain compounds that prevent bacteria from adhering to bladder walls, where they can lead to UTIs. (Blueberries will also do the trick.) If you are prone to UTIs, drink up. But also be sure to down plenty of water, which will help to flush harmful bacteria out of your system.

I've been treated for cystitis several times, but the symptoms never seem to go away completely. What's wrong?

It could be that you never completely eradicated the bacteria that are causing the problem. Never drink alcohol while on antibiotics, and always finish any antibiotic your doctor prescribes or the bug can come back with a vengeance. A new home test kit for UTIs can help you determine how well your drug regimen worked. It tests for the presence of the most common UTI-related bacteria. Called UTI, the test is available at many drugstores for about $10 (six tests included).

It's also possible that you have a more serious condition such as interstitial cystitis, in which the bladder wall is sensitive and feels full even when it is empty, or urethral diverticulum, a defect in the urethral "tube" that may produce a wide variety of symptoms—from incontinence to painful intercourse. If you suspect that either condition is to blame for your discomfort, consult with a doctor.

What does it mean if I wet myself when I cough or sneeze?

This is a symptom of stress incontinence, which results from a weakening of the muscles around the urethra. Sneezing, coughing, exercising, and even laughing can cause the bladder to leak urine.

Stress incontinence sometimes results from the strain of a vaginal childbirth, which weakens the pelvic-floor muscles and ligaments, leaving the urethra and bladder neck inadequately supported. The condition may worsen after menopause because the decline in hormones further weakens the pelvic-floor muscles. Smoking, obesity, and chronic constipation can increase the risk for stress incontinence. The treatment includes several self-help measures and, in extreme cases, corrective surgery.

How can I get incontinence under control?

Luckily there are several things you can do to control incontinence. Up to 70 percent of patients who suffer from mild to moderate stress incontinence can benefit from the following behavior modifications:

- Limit your intake of water to eight glasses a day. Avoid beverages that stimulate bladder contractions, such as alcohol and caffeinated drinks.
- Retrain your bladder by keeping track of when you urinate and how much urine you pass; then urinate on a schedule at regular intervals. Slowly lengthen the intervals to encourage your bladder to hold more urine.
- Strengthen the pelvic floor muscles by performing Kegels, simple clench-and-release exercises of the muscles you use to stop the urine stream. Tampon-shaped vaginal cones, called FemTone Vaginal Weights ($100–125), available without a prescription at drugstores, can also help by exercising the pelvic muscles with the added benefit of giving you clear signs of progress.
- Ask your doctor about prescription remedies, including antispasmodic medications, that relax the bladder and reduce contractions.

Breast Health

How can I make sure that I'm getting the best mammogram possible?
- Refrain from using deodorants, lotions, and powders on the skin near your breasts or under your arms before testing. These substances can obscure the mammogram.
- Make sure that the facility reading your mammogram has previous X rays with which to compare your test. This will provide a baseline for observing changes over time.
- If you have not heard from the mammography center or your physician within two weeks, call and request the results of your test. Don't assume that things are normal if you are not notified.

I took birth control pills for ten years. Does that increase my risk for breast cancer?

Probably not. Researchers recently took a thorough and thoughtful second look at fifty-four different studies to try to answer questions about pill use and breast cancer risk. The new study found that ten years after going off birth control pills, women who had used them were at no greater risk of breast cancer than women who had not. It didn't matter what the woman's age was when she started and stopped the Pill, the number of years on it, whether she had a family history of breast cancer, or the type or dose of pill used.

What can I do to reduce my risk of breast cancer?

Plenty. Only 25 percent of breast cancer cases are associated with risk factors out of a woman's control, such as a family history of the disease or early menstruation. That leaves a lot of room for effective behavioral changes.

- Limit your alcohol intake to one drink or less daily.
- Eat foods that are low in fat and high in fiber. Increase your intake of so-called cruciferous vegetables, such as broccoli and cauliflower, as well as food products made with soybeans.
- Exercise regularly. Research indicates that you can lower your risk by 40 to 50 percent with as little as four hours of mildly vigorous exercise weekly.
- Stay slim. Your risk increases proportionally as you gain weight.

Occasionally I notice some discharge from my breast. Should I worry?

Probably not. The mammary ducts collect a small amount of fluid that can be expressed if the breasts are manipulated. If the discharge is bloody, you should see a doctor at once because that may signal a more serious problem, such as breast cancer.

From time to time, both breasts may spontaneously emit a milky discharge, probably due to high levels of a hormone called prolactin, which is responsible for triggering the production of breast milk. Certain medications, including birth control pills, can also spike prolactin.

Menstrual Health

I was told I can't get pregnant while I'm having my period. Is this true?

No. While it's unlikely that you will get pregnant during menstruation, it is not impossible. To avoid pregnancy, you must use a reliable birth control method each time you have intercourse—even during your period.

I sometimes bleed slightly between my periods. What's wrong?

It's possible that nothing is wrong. Some women experience breakthrough bleeding (bleeding between periods) as a normal part of ovulation. Breakthrough bleeding is a common side effect with the IUD and hormonal methods of birth control, including the Pill, the mini-pill, and Norplant. If you are on the Pill and the problem continues for more than three months, speak to your health-care provider about trying a different formulation.

More serious causes of breakthrough bleeding include endometriosis, ectopic pregnancy, pelvic inflammatory disease, or cancer. If the problem continues, it's wise to see a doctor.

I'm on birth control pills and recently had some breakthrough bleeding after I started taking a drug for migraines. Can I get pregnant?

It's possible. If your migraine drug contains barbiturates, it may diminish the effectiveness of oral contraceptives. These drugs include Fiorinal and Fioricet. Other drugs that can compromise the Pill include certain antibiotics, anticonvulsant drugs like Tegretol and Dilantin, which are often prescribed for epilepsy, the tuberculosis drug rifampin, and certain antifungal medications. You may need to use a backup method of birth control while on these drugs to be on the safe side. Always remind your health-care provider that you are taking oral contraceptives when he gives you a prescription.

Why would my periods stop?

A wide range of factors can cause you to miss a period, including pregnancy. (A pregnancy test will help you rule out that possibility.) You can also miss a period if you are unusually stressed, if you have crossed several time zones (which interferes with the body's natural rhythms), or if you are taking certain medications, such as corticosteroids.

If you miss more than one period, you probably need to see a doctor to determine the cause. Several health conditions such as premature menopause, hypothyroidism, and eating disorders can cause menstrual periods to cease. For instance, women who have anorexia nervosa often lose so much body fat that their estrogen production is disrupted, halting ovulation. Excessive exercise can also interfere with hormone production. Any condition that stops ovulation can increase your risk for the bone-thinning disease osteoporosis.

How can I deal with my killer cramps?

Severe menstrual pain calls for serious medicine. You may find the best relief with drugs that target the culprits primarily responsible for menstrual discomfort, chemicals called prostaglandins. The most effective antiprostaglandin medications are Anaprox, Naprosyn, Ponstel, and Motrin.

Home remedies can also ease your suffering: taking hot baths, exercising, eating a balanced diet, and increasing your intake of vitamins and minerals—in particular, calcium, potassium, and magnesium.

My periods are getting more and more painful. What can I do?

It's probably wise to speak to your doctor to rule out a serious problem like endometriosis, which can affect your fertility. Endometriosis is sometimes signaled by menstrual pain that worsens over time or by pain during intercourse. It happens when the lining of the uterus—the endometrium—grows outside the uterus on other organs. During the menstrual period, the tissue bleeds just like the tissue inside the uterus, causing pain and scarring. If the endometriosis is not treated, the scarring can damage the reproductive organs, diminishing fertility.

Doctors typically treat endometriosis with hormones like those found in birth control pills, which suppress ovarian function. Surgery may be performed to remove the displaced endometrial tissue. In rare cases, the uterus is removed to stop ovulation altogether.

PMS turns me into a complete monster. What can I do?

There are many things you can do, depending on your symptoms:

- Reconsider your premenstrual menu. Consume plenty of complex carbohydrates and protein, and avoid salt, fat, caffeine, and alcohol.
- Take a vitamin B_6 supplement. (Don't exceed 150 mg. daily.)
- Exercise. Regular physical activity helps ease cramping, and aerobic exercise releases mood-elevating endorphins, which counteract depression.
- Ask your doctor about mood-enhancing drugs. Physicians are successfully treating premenstrual symptoms with the class of antidepressants known as selective serotonin reuptake inhibitors or SSRIs. Prozac, Paxil, and Zoloft are three of the SSRIs that may help regulate serotonin and thus help reduce mood-related symptoms.
- Try alternative remedies. Some women find relief with alternative therapies like acupuncture and relaxation techniques like yoga, meditation, and biofeedback.
- Consider herbs. Valerian root, hops, and passion flower may calm the nervous system. Parsley, dandelion, and sarsaparilla appear to

decrease water retention. Black cohosh, black hawk, and white willow bark can quell pain.

Menopause

I'm forty-one, and my periods have become wildly erratic. What gives?

You are probably experiencing perimenopause, or what doctors frequently call "the transition," the time period between normal menstruation and the cessation of monthly periods, says Donna Shoupe, M.D., professor of obstetrics and gynecology at the University of Southern California School of Medicine. It usually occurs between the ages of forty-five and fifty-five, and it lasts for approximately four years.

Perimenopause is often characterized by erratic hormone surges that result in irregular periods and abnormal bleeding. Women may also get hot flashes and flushes, insomnia, vaginal dryness, and a worsening of PMS symptoms.

Taking estrogen or starting HRT can help relieve the symptoms if they severely disrupt the quality of life. Some women in perimenopause go on oral contraceptives to regulate their periods.

Ever since I hit menopause, I've lost interest in sex. What can I do?

Consider hormone replacement therapy. After menopause, the vaginal walls tend to become thinner and drier in the absence of estrogen, which can make sex painful. Anticipating painful sex can diminish a woman's interest in it. If you are not taking estrogen, you may wish to speak to your doctor about starting it, or if you are already on it, about upping the dose.

Some doctors also prescribe testosterone, the primary sex-drive hormone, to women in menopause. Like estrogen, testosterone levels dip as the ovaries cease functioning, lowering libido in some women.

How can I deal with vaginal dryness?

The first thing to do is to let your doctor in on the problem. Hormone replacement therapy is the best way to deal with many of the symptoms of menopause, including vaginal dryness. Unfortunately, many patients do not get adequate relief from the regimens they practice. Adjusting the dose of estrogen (under a doctor's guidance) can sometimes help. For a quick fix, try an over-the-counter vaginal moisturizer or lubricant.

Women's Health Resources

American College of Obstetricians and Gynecologists
409 Twelfth Street, SW
Washington, DC 20024-2188
202-863-2518
(Free patient information)

American Social Health Association
Box 13827
Research Triangle Park, NC 27709
919-361-8400

Endometriosis Association
8585 North Seventy-sixth Place
Milwaukee, WI 53223
414-355-2200 or 1-800-992-3636

Hysterectomy Educational Resources
    and Services Foundation (HERS)
422 Bryn Mawr Avenue
Bala Cynwyd, PA 19004
610-667-7757

Institute for Research on Women's Health
1616 Eighteenth Street, NW, Suite 109B
Washington, DC 20009
202-483-8643

Interstitial Cystitis Association
Box 1553
Madison Square Station
New York, NY 10159
212-979-6057

Jacobs Institute of Women's Health
409 Twelfth Street, SW
Washington, DC 20024-2188
202-863-4990

Menopause Institute for Women's Health Research
1010 University Avenue
St. Paul, MN 55104
612-642-1951

Mid-life Women's Network
5129 Logan Avenue South
Minneapolis, MN 55419
800-886-4354

National Abortion Federation
1436 U Street, NW, Suite 103
Washington, DC 20009
202-667-5881

National Alliance of Breast Cancer Organizations
9 East Thirty-seventh Street, 10th Floor
New York, NY 10016
800-719-9154

National Asian Women's Health Organization
250 Montgomery Street, Suite 410
San Francisco, CA 94104
415-989-9747

National Association of Anorexia Nervosa and Associated Disorders (ANAD)
Box 7
Highland Park, IL 60035
847-831-3438 or 847-432-8000

National Association for Continence
P.O. Box 8310
Spartanburg, SC 29305
800-BLADDER (800-252-3337)

National Black Women's Health Project (NBWHP)
1237 Ralph David Abernathy Boulevard, SW
Atlanta, GA 30310
800-ASK-BWHP (800-275-2947)

National Kidney Foundation/UTI
Dept. UTI
30 E. Thirty-third Street
New York, NY 10016
212-889-2210

National Vulvodynia Association
P.O. Box 19288
Sarasota, FL 34276
941-927-8503

National Women's Health Network
514 Tenth Street, NW, Suite 400
Washington, DC 20004
202-347-1140

National Women's Health Resource Center
2425 L Street, NW, 3rd Floor
Washington, DC 20037
202-293-6045

Native American Women's Health Education Resource Center
P.O. Box 572
Lake Andes, SD 57356
605-487-7072

Planned Parenthood Federation of America
810 Seventh Avenue
New York, NY 10019
212-541-7800 or 800-230-7526 or 800-829-7732

RESOLVE, Inc. (Infertility information)
1310 Broadway
Somerville, MA 02144-1731
617-623-1156

Susan G. Komen Breast Cancer Foundation
5005 LBJ Freeway
Suite 370
Dallas, TX 57244
800-Im-Aware (462-9273)

Vulvar Pain Foundation
P.O. Drawer 177
Graham, NC 27253
910-226-0704

Y-Me National Breast Cancer Organization
212 West Van Buren, 5th Floor
Chicago, IL 60607
800-221-2141

Women and AIDS Resource Network (WARN)
30 Third Avenue, Suite 513
Brooklyn, NY 11217
718-596-6007

Hot Lines and Referral Services

American Cancer Society
800-ACS-2345

ASHA/CDC National STD Hotline
800-227-8922 (Monday–Friday, 8 A.M.–11 P.M., ET)
800-243-7012 (TTY/TDD)

CDC National AIDS Clearinghouse
800-458-5231

Eating Disorders Awareness and Prevention
206-382-3587

Emergency Contraception Hotline
888-NOT-TOO-LATE (888-668-2528)

National Abortion Federation Hotline
800-772-9100

National AIDS Hotline
800-342-AIDS (800-342-2437) (7 days/week, 24 hours/day)
Spanish Service:
800-344-7432 (7 days/week, 8 A.M. to 2 A.M., ET)
TTY for the Deaf (Monday to Friday, 8 A.M. to 2 A.M., ET):
800-243-7889

National Association of Anorexia Nervosa
    and Associated Disorders (ANAD) Hotline
847-831-3438

National Domestic Abuse Hotline
800-799-SAFE (800-799-7233)
800-787-3224 (TDD)

National Ovarian Cancer Coalition
888-OVARIAN (888-682-7426)

National Cancer Institute
Information Service
800-4-CANCER (800-422-6237)

PMS-Access
800-222-4767 (information)
800-558-7046 (physician referrals)

Selected Web Sites

Women's Health Issues
www.asa.ugl.lib.umich.edu/chdocs/womenhealth/womens_health.html
Guide to myriad women's health issues.

Women's Medical Health Page
www.best.com/~sirlou/wmhp.html
More women's health.

General Women's Health
www.thrive.com
Excellent source of women's health information.

Endometriosis Information and Links
www.ivf.com/witsend.html
In-depth information on dealing with endometriosis.

The Pap Test
www.erinet.com/fnadoc/pap.htm
A guide to understanding the Pap test.

Gyn 101: How to Ace Your Gynecological Exam
www.gyn101.com
A step-by-step guide to the gynecological exam and sexual health information.

S.P.O.T. The Tampon Health Website
www.critpath.org/~tracy/spot.html
Information on toxic shock syndrome and other potential dangers of tampons and other menstrual products.

Community Breast Health Project
www~med.stanford.edu/CBHP/

Duke University Women's Health Page
http://h-devil-www.mc.duke.edu/h-devil/women/women.htm

General Health Web Sites

www.healthfinder.gov
The U.S. government's site features health Web sites it has evaluated for accuracy and timeliness.

Planned Parenthood on the Web
www.ppfa.org
Basic reproductive health information.

Cancer Care Inc
www.cancercareinc.org
Offers on-line support groups for breast and gynecological cancer victims and family members.

Stork Site

www.storksite.com

A general pregnancy and parenting site.

The International Council for Infertility Information Dissemination (ICIID)

www.inciid.org

The ICIID site provides information on the diagnosis, treatment, and prevention of infertility and pregnancy loss.

Bibliography

Adelson, Joseph. "Sex Among the Americans." *Commentary* (July 1995): pp. 26–30.

Adler, T. "Family Planning Gets a Shot in the Arm." *Science News* (3 September 1994): p. 151.

Albert, Alexa E., David Lee Warner, Robert A. Hatcher, M.D., James Trussell, and Charles Bennett, M.D. "Condom Use Among Female Commercial Sex Workers in Nevada's Legal Brothels." *American Journal of Public Health* (November 1995): vol. 85, no. 11, p. 514.

Aldhous, Peter. "A Booster for Contraceptive Vaccines." *Science* (2 December 1994): vol. 266, pp. 1484–88.

Altman, Lawrence K. "With AIDS Advance, More Disappointment." *The New York Times* (19 January 1997): pp. A1, A14.

Ammer, Christine. *The New A to Z of Women's Health.* New York: Facts on File, 1995.

Angier, Natalie. "Illuminating How Bodies Are Built for Sociability." *The New York Times* (30 August 1996): p. C1.

Archer, David, F., Christine K. Mauck, Amabel Viniegra-Sibal, and Freedolph D. Anderson. "Lea's Shield®: A Phase 1 Postcoital Study of a New Contraceptive Barrier Device." *Contraception* (1995): vol. 52, pp. 167–73.

Asnes, Marion. "Birth Control Over 30." *Working Woman* (July 1994): pp. 68–72, 84.

Austin, Elizabeth. "How to Make Love to an Impotent Man." *American Health for Women* (November 1996): pp. 66–69.

Baron-Faust, Rita. "Welcome to Perimenopause: Life in Hormonal Limbo." *American Health for Women* (January/February 1997): pp. 70–73, 106.

Beazlie, Frank S., Jr., M.D. "Coital Injuries of Genitalia." *Medical Aspects of Human Sexuality* (August 1981): vol. 15, no. 8, pp. 112–21

Bechtel, Stefan. *The Sex Encyclopedia.* New York: Simon and Schuster, 1993.

Bechtel, Stefan, Laurence Roy Stains, and the editors of Men's Health Books. *Sex: A Man's Guide.* Emmaus, Penn. Rodale Press, 1996.

Beitiks, Edvins. "Celestial Seasonings: The Fine Art of Wooing with Food and Drink." *San Francisco Examiner* (8 February 1995): p. Z1.

Belk, Jan. "The Good Doctor." *Salisbury Post* (N.C.) (9 December 1990): pp. C1, C13.

Berendt, John. "The Orgasm Reconsidered." *Esquire* (June 1993): pp. 27–29.

Blakeslee, Sandra. "2 New Treatments for Erectile Ills." *The New York Times* (9 August 1995): p. C8.

Bone, Eugenia. "When You Don't Pass Your Pap Test." *Mademoiselle* (April 1996): p. 104.

Boodman, Sandra G. "Emergency Contraception." *Washington Post* (4 April 1995): Health sec., p. 7.

The Boston Women's Health Book Collective. *The New Our Bodies, Ourselves.* New York: Simon and Schuster, 1994.

Bower, B. "Nice Guys Look Better in Women's Eyes." *Science News* (18 March 1995): p. 165.

"Breast Lumps: What to Do If You Find One." *Mayo Clinic Health Letter* (April 1997): vol. 15, no. 4, p. 4.

"British Pill Scare Leaves American Women Unfazed." *Contraceptive Technology Update*® (January 1996): pp. 6, 7, 9–10.

Britton, Bryce, and Stephen Kiesling. "The Little Muscle That Matters." *American Health* (September 1986): pp. 59–61.

Brodey, Denise. "A User's Guide to the Pill." *Mademoiselle* (April 1995): p. 112.

Brody, Jane E. "A New Look at an Old Quest for Sexual Stimulants" (Personal Health Column). *The New York Times* (4 August 1993): p. C12.

———. "With More Help Available for Impotence, Few Men Seek It" (Personal Health Column). *The New York Times* (2 August 1995): p. C9.

———. "Impotence: More Options, More Experts, More Success." (Personal Health Column). *The New York Times* (9 August 1995) p. C8.

Brownlee, Shannon. "Can't Do Without Love: What Science Says About Those Tender Feelings." *US News & World Report* (17 February 1997): vol. 122, no. 6, pp. 58–61.

Bryan, Toni. "There Can Be Sexual Anorexia Too." *Cosmopolitan* (November 1993): pp. 101–102.

Busby, Trent, M.D. *Be Good to Your Body.* Secaucus, N.J.: The Citadel Press, 1976.

Cadoff, Jennifer. "What You Need to Know to Get the Best Possible Pap Smear and to Make Optimal Treatment Choices If You're One of the Many Women Who Will Be Faced with an Abnormal Result." *Glamour* (March 1993): pp. 212–16.

Carey, Michael P., and Blair T. Johnson. "Effectiveness of Yohimbine in the Treatment of Erectile Disorder: Four Meta-Analytic Integrations." *Archives of Sexual Behavior* (August 1996): vol. 25, no. 4, pp. 341–61.

Carlson, Karen J., M.D., Stephanie Eisenstat, M.D., and Terra Ziporyn. *The Harvard Guide to Women's Health.* Cambridge: Harvard University Press, 1995.

"Cervical Cytology: Evaluation and Management of Abnormalities." *ACOG Technical Bulletin* (August 1993): no. 183.

Chalker, Rebecca. "Sexual Pleasure Unscripted." *Ms.* (November/December 1995): pp. 49–52.

Chia, Mantak, and Douglas Abrams Arava. *The Multi-Orgasmic Man.* San Francisco: Harper, 1996.

Chrisler, Joan C., Ingrid K. Johnston, Nicole M. Champagne, and Kathleen E. Preston. "Menstrual Joy: The Construct and Its Consequences." *Psychology of Women Quarterly* (1994): vol. 18, pp. 375–87.

Christina, Greta. "Are We Having Sex Yet?" *Ms.* (November/December 1995): pp. 60–62.

"Clarification: Cervical Cancer Screening Devices." *National Women's Health Report* (August 1996): vol. 18, no. 4, p. 6.

Cohen, Patricia. "The IUD: Birth-Control Device That the U.S. Market Won't Bear." *Washington Post* (6 August 1996): p. A1.

Colino, Stacey. "The Bloat Report." *Self* (November 1994): pp. 88–89.

Collins, and Huntley. "U.S. Guidelines Say Doctors Should Urge Pregnant Women with HIV to Use AZT." *Knight-Ridder/Tribune News Service* (9 August 1994).

"Contraceptive Use." *Facts in Brief.* New York: The Alan Guttmacher Institute (4 January 1993).

"Contraceptives and Other Reproductive Health Products Under Development by The Population Council." (Report) New York: The Population Council, December 1995.

"Contraceptives: What's New, What's Coming Up." *Glamour* (October 1993): p. 84.

Cotton, Paul. "How 'Definitive' Is New Sex Survey? Answers Vary." *Journal of the American Medical Association* (14 December 1994): vol. 272, no. 22, p. 1727.

Craze, Richard. *The Spiritual Traditions of Sex.* New York: Crown Publishers, 1996.

Crenshaw, Theresa L., M.D. *The Alchemy of Love and Lust.* New York: G. P. Putnam, 1996.

Curtis, Tom. "The Female Condom." *Self* (April 1993): pp. 138–41, 176–79.

Darling, Carol Anderson, J. Kenneth Davidson, Sr., and Colleen Conway-Welch. "Female Ejaculation: Perceived Origins, the Grafenberg Spot/Area, and Sexual Responsiveness." *Archives of Sexual Behavior* (1990): vol. 19, no. 1, pp. 29–47.

Darling, Carol Anderson, J. Kenneth Davidson, Sr., and Donna A. Jennings. "The Female Sexual Response Revisited: Understanding the Multiorgasmic Experience in Women." *Archives of Sexual Behavior,* (1991): vol. 20, no. 6, pp. 527–40.

Davidson, J. Kenneth, Sr., and Carol Anderson Darling. "Self-Perceived Differences in the Female Orgasmic Response." *Family Practice Research Journal* (1989): vol. 8, pp. 75–84.

———. "The Stereotype of Single Women Revisited: Sexual Practices and Sexual Satisfaction Among Professional Women." *Health Care for Women International* (1988): vol. 9, pp. 317–36.

Davidson, J. Kenneth, Sr., Carol A. Darling, and Colleen Conway-Welch. "The Role of the Grafenberg Spot and Female Ejaculation in the Female Orgasmic Response: An Empirical Analysis." *Journal of Sex & Marital Therapy* (Summer 1989): vol. 15, no. 2, pp. 102–20.

DeBlieu, January "It's a Crime." *Health* (July/August 1996): pp. 83–87.

Delaney, Janice, Mary Jane Lupton, and Emily Toth. *The Curse: A Cultural History of Menstruation.* Urbana, Ill.: University of Illinois Press, 1988

DeNoon, Daniel J. "Protease Inhibitors: The Good and the Bad." *AIDS Weekly Plus* (19 August 1996): pp. 3–6.

Doskoch, Peter. "The Safest Sex." *Psychology Today* (September/October 1995): pp. 46–49.

"Doublechecking Pap Smears." *FDA Consumer* (March 1996): p. 3.

Drexler, Madeline. "What Can You Do About Endometriosis?" *Self* (January 1995): pp. 122–23, 139.

———. "Facts About Your Period." *Self* (February 1995): pp. 76–77.

Dugger, Celia W. "Woman's Plea for Asylum Puts Tribal Ritual on Trial." *The New York Times* (15 April 1996): p. A1.

———. "U.S. Hearing to Decide Rights of Women Who Flee Genital Mutilation." *The New York Times* (2 May 1996): p. B6.

Ebi, Kristie L., Robert L. Piziali, Michael Rosenberg, and Harry F. Wachob. "Evidence Against Tailstrings Increasing the Rate of Pelvic Inflammatory Disease Among IUD Users." *Contraception* (1996): vol. 53, pp. 25–32.

Ellertson, Charlotte. "History and Efficacy of Emergency Contraception: Beyond Coca-Cola." *Family Planning Perspectives* (March/April 1996): vol. 28, no. 2, pp. 44–48.

Ellis, Bruce J., and Donald Symons. "Sex Differences in Sexual Fantasy: An Evolutionary Psychological Approach." *The Journal of Sex Research* (November 1990): vol. 27, no. 4, pp. 527–55.

"Empower Your Patients by Teaching Genital Self-Exam." *Contraceptive Technology Update®* (June 1995): pp. 73–74.

Endicott, Jean, Ellen W. Freeman, Andrea M. Kielich, M.D., and Steven J. Sond-heimer, M.D. "PMS: New Treatments That Really Work." *Patient Care* (15 April 1996): pp. 88–119.

Eng, Thomas R., and William T. Butler, eds. "The Hidden Epidemic: Confronting Sexually Transmitted Diseases." (Institute of Medicine) Washington, D.C.: National Academy Press, 1996.

"Epidemic Growing Among Women." *AIDS Alert* (June 1996): vol. 11, no. 6, pp. 71–73.

"Experimental Treatment Access for Women with HIV Demanded." *AIDS Weekly* (3 October 1994): pp. 11–12.

"Family Planners: Beware 'Lunatic Fringe Sperm.'" *Contraceptive Technology Up-date*® (June 1995): p. 71.

Farr, Gaston, Henry Gabelnick, Kim Sturgen, and Laneta Dorflinger. "Contracep-tive Efficacy and Acceptability of the Female Condom." *American Journal of Public Health* (December 1994): vol. 84, no. 12, pp. 1960–64.

"Fathering Healthy Babies." *University of California at Berkeley Wellness Letter* (April 1994): vol. 10, issue 7, pp. 1–2.

The Federation of Feminist Health Centers. *The New View of a Woman's Body.* Los Angeles: Feminist Health Press, 1995.

"Fertility, Family Planning, and Women's Health: New Data from the 1995 Na-tional Survey of Family Growth." U.S. Department of Health and Human Ser-vices, *DHHS Publication No. (PHS) 97–1995*, series 23, no. 19.

Finn, Stephen D., Edward J. Boyko, Esther H, Normand, Chi-Ling Chen, Jane R. Grafton, Marcia Hunt, Patricia Yarbro, Delia Scholes, and Andy Stergachis. "Association Between Use of Spermicide-Coated Condoms and *Escherichia coli* Urinary Tract Infection in Young Women." *American Journal of Epidemiol-ogy* (1998): vol. 144, no. 6, pp. 512–20.

Forrest, Jacqueline Darroch. "Contraceptive Use in the United States: Past, Present and Future." *Advances in Population* (1994): vol. 2, pp. 29–48.

————. "Epidemiology of Unintended Pregnancy and Contraceptive Use." *Ameri-can Journal of Obstetrics and Gynecology* (May 1994): vol. 170, no. 5, part 2, pp. 1485–89.

Furlow, F. Bryant. "The Smell of Love." *Psychology Today* (March/April 1996): pp. 38–45.

Furlow, F. Bryant, and Randy Thornhill. "The Orgasm Wars." *Psychology Today* (January/February 1996): pp. 42–46.

Gabbay, Mark, and Alan Gibbs. "Does Additional Lubrication Reduce Condom Failure?" *Contraception* (1996): vol. 53, pp. 155–58.

Geerling, John H. "Natural Family Planning." *American Family Physician* (1 No-vember 1995): vol. 52, no. 6, pp. 1749–1759.

Geller, Zoë. "Tools for Love: AKA Sex Toys." *Cosmopolitan* (March 1996): pp. 156–58.

Gelsanter, Carey Quan. "Urinary Tract Infections." *Seattle Times* (19 February 1997): pp. E1, E5.

Gianelli, Diane M. "Fertility Scandal Raises Call for Regulation." *American Medical News* (11 September 1995): pp. 3, 29.

———. "Fertility Clinic: Baby in Three Tries or Your Money Back." *American Medical News* (25 September 1995): p. 4.

Goleman, Daniel. "Sex Fantasy Research Said to Neglect Women." *The New York Times* (14 June 1995): sec. C, p. 14.

Goodman, Susan. "Sexual Fitness." *Redbook* (October 1995): pp. 96–99.

Graves, Ginny. "Exercises for Great Sex." *Self* (April 1995): p. 78.

Grodstein, Francine, Meir J. Stampfer, Graham A. Colditz, Walter C. Willett, JoAnn E. Manson, Marshall Joffe, Bernard Rosner, Charles Fuchs, Susan E. Hankinson, David J. Hunter, Charles H. Hennekens, and Frank E. Speizer. "Postmenopausal Hormone Therapy and Mortality." *New England Journal of Medicine* (19 June 1997): vol. 336, no. 25, pp. 1769–75.

Hagan, Carolyn P. "Brave New Checkup." *Mademoiselle* (June 1995): pp. 80–82.

———. "When Your Period Is Weird." *Mademoiselle* (May 1996): pp. 104–106.

Hanrahan, Susan Noll. "Historical Review of Menstrual Toxic Shock Syndrome." *Women & Health* (1994): vol. 21 (2/3), pp. 141–65.

Harris, Lynn. "Making Love Better." *Ladies' Home Journal* (July 1995): pp. 48, 54–56.

Harrison, Polly F., and Allan Rosenfield, eds. "Contraceptive Research and Development: Looking to the Future." (Institute of Medicine) Washington, D.C.: National Academy Press, 1996.

Hatcher, Robert A., M.D. James Trussell, Felicia Stewart, M.D., Gary K. Stewart, M.D., Deborah Kowal, Felicia Guest, Willard Cates, Jr., M.D., and Michael S. Policar, M.D. *Contraceptive Technology.* New York: Irvington Publishers 1994.

Hatcher, Robert A., M.D., James Trussell, Felicia Stewart, M.D., Susan Howells, Caroline R. Russell, and Deborah Kowal. *Emergency Contraception: The Nation's Best-Kept Secret.* Atlanta, Ga.: Bridging the Gap Communications, 1995.

Hawes, Stephen E., Sharon L. Hillier, Jacqueline Benedetti, Claire E. Stevens, Laura A. Koutsky, Pål Wølner-Hanssen, and King K. Holmes. "Hydrogen Peroxide-Producing Lactobacilli and Acquisition of Vaginal Infections." *The Journal of Infectious Diseases* (1996): vol. 174, pp. 1058–63.

"Health Maintenance for Perimenopausal Women." *ACOG Technical Bulletin* (August 1995): no. 210.

Heise, Lori, Kirsten Moore, and Nahid Toubia. *Sexual Coercion and Reproductive Health: A Focus on Research.* New York: The Population Council, 1995.

Herman, Robin. "Whatever Happened to the Contraceptive Revolution?" *The Washington Post* (13 December 1994): p. 13.

Hogshire, Jim. "Take Two and See Me in the Morning." *GQ* (July 1995): vol. 65, no. 7, pp. 62–63.

Hooton, Thomas M., Delia Scholes, James P. Hughes, Carol Winter, Pacita L. Roberts, Ann E. Stapleton, Andy Stergachis, and Walter E. Stamm. "A Prospective Study of Risk Factors for Symptomatic Urinary Tract Infection in Young Women." *New England Journal of Medicine* (15 August 1996): vol. 335, no. 7, pp. 468–74.

"Hormonal Contraception." *ACOG Technical Bulletin* (October 1994): no. 198.

"Hormone Therapy: How to Manage Side Effects." *Women's Health Advocate Newsletter* (January 1997): vol. 3, no. 11, pp. 4–5.

"Hormone Therapy: When and for How Long?" *Health News* (from the publisher of *New England Journal of Medicine*) (25 March 1997): vol. 3, no. 4, pp. 1–2.

"How to Decipher Your Pap Results." *Women's Health Advocate Newsletter* (April 1997): vol. 4, no. 2, p. 7.

Hurlbert, David Farley, and Carol Apt. "The Coital Alignment Technique and Directed Masturbation: A Comparative Study on Female Orgasm." *Journal of Sex & Marital Therapy* (Spring 1995): vol. 21, no. 1, pp. 21–29.

Hurlbert, David Farley, and Karen Elizabeth Whittaker. "The Role of Masturbation in Marital and Sexual Satisfaction: A Comparative Study of Female Masturbators and Nonmasturbators." *Journal of Sex Education and Therapy* (1991): vol. 17, no. 4, pp. 272–82.

"In Search of the Fountain of Youth—Hormone Replacement Therapy." *Lifetime Health Letter* (The University of Texas—Houston Health Science Center) (January 1997): vol. 9. no. 1, pp. 6–7.

Indian Council of Medical Research Task Force on Natural Family Planning. "Field Trial of Billings Ovulation Method of Natural Family Planning." *Contraception* (1996): vol. 53, pp. 69–74.

Ingall, Marjorie. "S-E-X in the U.S.A. Wake Us When It's Over." *Ms.* (January/February 1995): p. 93.

Jacobowitz, Ruth S. *150 Most-Asked Questions About Midlife Sex, Love, and Intimacy.* New York: Hearst Books, 1995.

Jewelewicz, Raphael. "Natural Family Planning or Rhythm Method." *The Columbia University College of Physicians and Surgeons Complete Home Medical Guide, Edition 2.* New York: Crown Publishers, 1989.

"The Kaiser Survey on Public Knowledge and Attitudes on Contraception and Unplanned Pregnancy 1995." Menlo Park, Calif.: The Henry J. Kaiser Family Foundation, 1995.

Kase, Lori Miller. "The Pill Is Safe." *Self* (April 1992): pp. 135, 192.

Katzman, Lisa. "X-tasy." *New Woman* (September 1994): pp. 113–15, 146.

Kearns, Michelle, and Valerie Frankel. "The Big O." *Redbook* (January 1992): pp. 55–57, 90.

Kelleher, Kathleen. "Odds of Conception May Be Better If Sex Is Good for Her." *Los Angeles Times* (19 February 1996): p. E3.

Kent, Debra. "What You Don't Know About Orgasm Could Thrill You." *Mademoiselle* (February 1990): pp. 154–55.

Keton, Jeannette S., and Tracy Chutorian Semler. "Is It PMS? PDD? Or Are You Just in a Really Bad Mood?" *Ladies' Home Journal* (October 1995): pp. 86, 88–89, 205.

Kistner, R. W. "Physiology of the Vagina." *The Human Vagina*. E. S. E. Hafez and T. N. Evans, eds. Amsterdam: Elsevier/North Holland Biomedical Press. 1978.

Kitasei, Hilary Hinds. "STDs: What You Don't Know Can Hurt You." *Ms.* (March/April 1995): pp. 24–29.

Kolata, Gina. "RU 486: It Isn't Just Popping a Pill." *The New York Times* (28 July 1996): p. E14.

Koontz, Katy. "Measure Your Contraception." *Glamour* (March 1996): pp. 224–25, 239–41.

Kotz, Deborah. "5 Questions You *Must* Ask Your Gynecologist." *McCall's* (October 1993): pp. 35–36.

Laan, Ellen, Walter Everaerd, Gerdy van Bellen, and Gerrit Hanewald. "Women's Sexual and Emotional Responses to Male- and Female-Produced Erotica." *Archives of Sexual Behavior* (1994): vol. 23, no. 2, pp. 153–61.

Ladas, A. K., B. Whipple, and J. D. Perry. *The G Spot and Other Recent Discoveries About Human Sexuality*. New York: Dell Publishers, 1983.

Lauersen, Neils, M.D., and Steven Whitney, with Eileen Stukane. *It's Your Body: A Woman's Guide to Gynecology*. New York: The Body Press/Perigee, 1993.

Laumann, Edward O., Robert T. Michael, and John H Gagnon. "A Political History of the National Sex Survey of Adults." *Family Planning Perspectives* (January/February 1994): vol. 26, no. 1, pp. 34–38.

Lawhead, R. Allen, Jr. M.D. "Vulvar Self-Examination: What Your Patients Should Know." *The Female Patient* (January 1990): vol. 15, pp. 33–34, 36, 38.

Legato, Marianne J., M.D. "Health Care in the United States: The New Focus on Women." *The Female Patient* (February Supplement 1995): pp. 33–39.

Lerner, Sharon. "Are the Treatment Options for PMS Leaving You Bloated, Irritable, and Crampy?" *Ms.* (July/August 1996): pp. 38–41.

Lever, Janet, and Pepper Schwartz. "Why Is Intercourse Painful for Her?" *Glamour* (April 1996): p. 87.

Levine, Judith. "Is Sex Natural?" *New Woman* (April 1996): pp. 92–96, 146.

Lewin, Tamar. "So, Now We Know What Americans Do in Bed. So?" *The New York Times* (9 October 1994): p. E3.

————. "F.D.A. Approval Sought for French Abortion Pill." *The New York Times* (1 April 1996): p. A8.

————. "U.S. Agency Wants the Pill Redefined." *The New York Times* (1 July 1996): pp. A1, B6.

Livermore, Beth. "Why Women's Orgasms Matter." *Self* (February 1994): p. 56.

"Love Hurts." *Men's Confidential Newsletter* (Rodale Press) (June 1994): pp. 1–2.

"Mammograms Under 50." *Consumer Reports on Health* (April 1997): vol. 9, no. 4, p. 44.

Mann, Klaus, M.D., Thomas Klingler, M.D., Susanne Noe, Joachim Röschke, M.D., Stefan Müller, M.D., and Otto Benkert, M.D. "Effects of Yohimbine on Sexual Experiences and Nocturnal Penile Tumescence and Rigidity in Erectile Dysfunction." *Archives of Sexual Behavior* (1996): vol. 25, no. 1, pp. 1–16.

Mayer, Ruth. "12 Ways Not to Get Pregnant." *Mademoiselle* (August 1993): pp. 194–95.

McCoy, Norma L., and Joseph R. Matyas. "Oral Contraceptives and Sexuality in University Women." *Archives of Sexual Behavior* (1996): vol. 25, no. 1, pp. 73–89.

"Medical Abortion With Mifepristone and Misoprostol." (Report.) New York: The Population Council September 1995.

Modahl, Charlotte. "The Love Hormone." *Mademoiselle* (November 1990): p. 112.

Monagle, Katie. "All About Eve's Garden." *Ms.* (November/December 1995): pp. 53–55.

Money, John. Review of *Sex in America: A Definitive Survey,* by Robert T. Michael, John H. Gagnon, Edward O. Laumann, and Gina Kolata. *The New England Journal of Medicine* (25 May 1995): pp. 1452–53.

Morgan, Peggy, Caroline Saucer, Elisabeth Torg, and the Editors of Prevention Magazine Health Books. *The Female Body: An Owner's Manual.* Emmaus, Penn.: Rodale Press, 1996.

Morokoff, Patricia J. "Sexuality in Perimenopausal and Postmenopausal Women." *Psychology of Women Quarterly* (1988): vol. 12, pp. 489–511.

Muir, Charles and Caroline. "Tantric Sex: The Art of Conscious Loving." *New Woman* (May 1990): pp. 106–109.

Murray, Linda. "Better Sex Through Chemistry." *Longevity* (August 1993): pp. 26, 66, 68.

"New Barrier Methods for Women in Development." *Contraceptive Technology Update*® (November 1994): p. 143.

"New Name, Treatments for Impotence." *HealthNews* (Massachussets Medical Society) (10 December 1996): p. 3.

"New Papanicolaou Test." *American Family Physician* (1 September 1996): p. 1121.

Nordenberg, TaMarch "The Facts About Aphrodisiacs." *FDA Consumer* (January/February 1996): vol. 30, no. 1, pp. 10–16.

Northrup, Christiane, M.D. *Women's Bodies, Women's Wisdom.* New York: Bantam Books, 1994.

O'Shaughnessy, Lynn. "The Ultimate Contraceptive." *Healthy Woman* (Winter 1995): pp. 20–21.

Ogden, Gina. "Hot Summer Nights: Want to Make Love Like You Used to?" *Ladies' Home Journal* (August 1995): vol. 112, no. 8, pp. 38–41.

The PDR Family Guide to Women's Health and Prescription Drugs. Montvale, N.J.: Medical Economics Data Production Co., 1994.

Padian, Nancy S., Stephen C. Shiboski, and Nicholas P. Jewell. "Female-to-Male Transmission of Human Immunodeficiency Virus." *Journal of the American Medical Association* (25 September 1991): vol. 266, no. 12, pp. 1664–67.

"Pap Smears & You: A Winning Team Against Cervical Cancer." *Johns Hopkins Women's Health* (September 1995): pp. 1, 3–5.

"Pap Smears: New Screening Methods Emerge; Do They Deliver as Promised?" *Women's Health Advocate Newsletter* (March 1997): vol. 4, no. 1, pp. 1, 6.

Parker, William H., M.D., with Rachel L. Parker. *A Gynecologist's Second Opinion.* New York: Plume/Penguin, 1996.

Pasquale, Samuel A., M.D., and Jennifer Cadoff. *The Birth Control Book.* New York: Ballantine Books, 1996.

Pechter, Kerry. "The Aphrodisiacs." *Men's Health* (Spring 1988): pp. 43–44.

Peters, Lynn. "The Best Position for Making Love (Hint: You Don't Have to Be on Top)." *Redbook* (February 1996): pp. 82–85.

Peterson, Herbert B., M.D., Zhisen Xia, Joyce M. Hughes, Lynne S. Wilcox, M.D., Lisa Ratliff Tylor, and James Trussell. "The Risk of Pregnancy After Tubal Sterilization: Findings from the U.S. Collaborative Review of Sterilization." *American Journal of Obstetrics and Gynecology* (April 1996): pp. 1161–70.

"Physicians Emphasize Availability of Emergency Oral Contraception." *ACOG News Release* (28 April 1997).

"The Pill: What We Know Now: Reconsidering Risks and Benefits." *Women's Health Advocate Newsletter* (June 1995): vol. 2, no. 4, pp. 1, 6.

The Planned Parenthood Women's Health Encyclopedia. New York: Crown Trade Paperbacks, 1996.

"The Politics of Masturbation." *The Lancet* (24/31 December 1994): vol. 344, pp. 1714–15.

Profet, Margie. "Menstruation As a Defense Against Pathogens Transported by Sperm." *The Quarterly Review of Biology* (September 1993): vol. 68, no. 3, pp. 335–37.

"Prostitutes Tell How to Improve Condom Use." *Contraceptive Technology Update*® (December 1995): pp. 150, 155.

Raab, Scott. "Love Hurts." *Self* (April 1994): pp. 110, 114.

"Recommendations on Frequency of Pap Test Screening." *ACOG Committee Opinion* (March 1995): no. 152.

Redmond, Geoffrey, M.D. *The Good News About Women's Hormones*. New York: Warner Books, 1995.

Reinisch, June M., dir. *The Kinsey Institute New Report on Sex*. New York: St. Martin's Press, 1991.

Rigby, Julie. "Oh! Oooh! Ewww! 7 Women Review the New Sex Movies." *Redbook* (October 1995): pp. 73–74.

Roberts, Claire. "When You've Lost That Loving Feeling . . ." *London Life* (20 December 1994): p. 32.

Roberts, Susan. "Revolutionary New Methods of Natural Birth Control." *Self* (October 1994): p. 72.

Rosen, Raymond C., Jennifer F. Taylor, Sandra R. Leiblum, and Gloria A. Bachmann. "Prevalence of Sexual Dysfunction in Women: Results of a Survey Study of 329 Women in an Outpatient Gynecological Clinic." *Journal of Sex and Marital Therapy* (Fall 1993): vol. 19, no. 3, pp. 171–88.

Rowland, David L., Khalid Kallan, and A. Koos Slob. "Yohimbine, Erectile Capacity, and Sexual Response in Men." *Archives of Sexual Behavior* (February 1997): vol. 26, no. 1, pp. 49–63.

Runowicz, Carolyn, M.D. "New Pap Test Technology." *HealthNews* (31 December 1996): p. 3.

Ryder, Bob, and Hubert Campbell. "Natural Family Planning in the 1990s." *The Lancet* (22 July 1995): vol. 346, no. 8969, pp. 233–35.

Sales, Nancy Jo. "How to Reach Sex Heaven on Earth." *Mademoiselle* (March 1996): pp. 156–59.

Scanlon, Deralee. "Oysters, Chocolate, Apricots as Aphrodisiacs: Fact or Fantasy?" *Environmental Nutrition* (June 1994): vol. 17, no. 6, pp. 1–2.

Schaff, Eric A., M.D., Steven H. Eisinger, M.D., Peter Franks, M.D., and Suzy S. Kim. "Methotrexate and Misoprostol for Early Abortion." *Family Medicine* (March 1996): vol. 28, no. 3, pp. 198–203.

Schwartz, Judith. "Can You Have a Better Orgasm?" *Redbook* (November 1994): pp. 96–97, 133.

Seaman, Barbara. *The Doctors' Case Against the Pill*. Alameda, Calif.: Hunter House, 1969.

Sedgwick, John "The Estrogen Report." *Self* (March 1994): pp. 133–35, 174–79.

———. "Beware of STDs." *Self* (July 1995): pp. 98–102, 139.

"Sexual Dysfunction." *ACOG Technical Bulletin* (September 1955): no. 211.

Snowden, Lynn. "The C Spot." *Self* (February 1993): pp. 134, 160–61.

Soderstrom, Richard M., M.D. "Latest Developments in Menstrual Protection." *Contemporary Ob/Gyn* (15 April 1996): pp. 91–100.

Spangler, Tina. "Natural Birth Control." *Natural Health* (September/October 1995): vol. 25, no. 5, pp. 42–46.

Sparkman, Robin. "Finally, a PMS Pill That Works." *Health* (November/December 1995): pp. 46–48.

"Special Report: Should You Be Tested for HIV? At Home?" *University of California at Berkeley Wellness Letter* (January 1997): vol. 13, issue 4, p. 4.

"Spermicide-Coated Condoms Boost Urinary Tract Infections." *AIDS Weekly Plus* (16 September 1996): pp. 20–22.

Squires, Sally. "Most Pregnancies Unplanned or Unwanted, Study Says." *The Washington Post* (9 May 1997): Health sec., p. 7.

Stenson, Jacqueline. "Emergency Contraception." *Self* (August 1995): p. 60.

Stewart, Felicia, M.D., Felicia Guest, Gary Stewart, M.D., and Robert Hatcher, M.D. *Understanding Your Body.* New York: Bantam Books, 1987.

Stoppard, Miriam, M.D. *The Magic of Sex.* New York: Dorling Kindersley, 1991.

"Study Details Sexuality in America." *Christian Century* (2 November 1994): pp. 1008–9.

"Survival of the Sexually Fit." *Men's Confidential Newsletter* (Rodale Press) (November 1994): pp. 11–12.

Taylor, Dena, and Sue Smith-Heavenrich. "The Power of Menstruation." *Mothering* (January 1991): pp. 10–16.

"Testosterone and HRT." *Women's Health Watch*™ (Harvard Medical School) (June 1996): vol. 3, no. 1, p. 1.

Thomas, Dana. "Anatomy of an Orgasm." *Self* (March 1992): pp. 113–17.

Trussell, James, "Contraceptive Efficacy." *Arch Dermatol* (September 1995): vol. 131, pp. 1064–68.

Trussell, James, Joseph A. Leveque, M.D., Jacqueline D. Koenig, Robert London, M.D., Spencer Borden, M.D., Joan Henneberry, Katherine D. LaGuardia, M.D., Felicia Stewart, M.D., T. George Wilson, M.D., Susan Wysocki, and Michael Strauss, M.D. "The Economic Value of Contraception: A Comparison of 15 Methods." *American Journal of Public Health* (April 1995): vol. 85, no. 4, pp. 494–503.

"Two New Surveys of American Public and Physicians." (News release.) Menlo Park, Calif.: The Henry J. Kaiser Family Foundation (29 March 1995).

Ulmann, André, Georges Teutsch, and Daniel Philibert. "RU 486." *Scientific American* (June 1990): vol. 262, no. 6, pp. 42–48.

"Understanding Breast Changes: A Health Guide for All Women." *NIH Publication no. 93-3536* (April 1993).

"U.S. Public Health Service Recommendations for Human Immunodeficiency Virus Counseling and Voluntary Testing for Pregnant Women." *CDC Prevention Guidelines* (7 July 1995): MMWR 44 (RR-7), pp. 1–15.

"Vagina Self-Exam Can Detect Cancer Early." Supplement to *Contraceptive Technology Update®* (May 1995): p. 1.

The Vaginal Infections and Prematurity Study Group. "Association Between Bacterial Vaginosis and Preterm Delivery of a Low-Birth-Weight Infant." *New England Journal of Medicine* (28 December 1995): vol. 333, no. 26, p. 1737.

Voigt, Harrison. "Enriching the Sexual Experience of Couples: The Asian Traditions and Sexual Counseling." *Journal of Sex and Marital Therapy* (Fall 1991): vol. 17, no. 3, pp. 214–19.

Walker, Morton, M.D. *Sexual Nutrition.* New York: Avery Publishing Group, 1994.

Walker, Richard. *The Family Guide to Sex and Relationships.* New York: Macmillan, 1996.

Weinhouse, Beth. "The Facts About Pap Smears." *Parents* (September 1995): pp. 35–39.

Weiss, Rick. "Prescription for Passion." *Health* (September 1995): vol. 9, no. 5, pp. 100–105.

Weschler, Toni. *Taking Care of Your Fertility.* New York: HarperPerennial, 1995.

Westheimer, Ruth K., with Joanne Serling. "Dr. Ruth's Reading List." *New Woman* (December 1993): pp. 50–53.

Whipple, Beverly. "Research Concerning Sexual Response in Women." *The Health Psychologist* (Fall 1995): vol. 17, no. 3, p. 16.

Whipple, Beverly, and Gina Ogden. *Safe Encounters: How Women Can Say Yes to Pleasure and No to Unsafe Sex.* New York: Pocket Books, 1990.

Whipple, Beverly, Gina Ogden, and Barry R. Komisaruk. "Physiological Correlates of Imagery-Induced Orgasm in Women." *Archives of Sexual Behavior* (1992): vol. 21, no. 2, pp. 121–33.

Winikoff, Beverly, M.D., and Suzanne Wymelenberg. *The Contraceptive Handbook.* Yonkers, N.Y.: Consumer Reports Books, 1992.

Winks, Cathy, and Ann Seamans. *The Good Vibrations Guide to Sex.* Pittsburgh: Cleis Press, 1994.

Winton, Mark A. "Editorial: The Social Construction of the G-Spot and Female Ejaculation." *Journal of Sex Education and Therapy* (1989): vol. 15, no. 3, pp. 151–62.

Wolff, Jennifer. "The Chemistry of Cramps." *Self* (February 1994): pp. 102–103.

Young Stephen. "The Subtle Side of Sex." *New Scientist* (14 August 1993): pp. 24–27.

Youngkin, Ellis Quinn, and Marcia Szamania Davis, eds. *Women's Health: A Primary Care Clinical Guide.* Norwalk, Conn.: Appleton and Lange, 1994.

Index